Praise for *Dying to Be a Good Mother*

"I very seldom meet such a wonderful survivor who says what she lived. Heather Chauvin's compelling story of loss and ultimate triumph is a testament to the power of the human spirit, and of celebrating both what remains, and what is found, after hitting rock bottom. Her warmth, wit, and shining example will help propel you forward to climb your way to your true self and decide to be the real you."

DR. EDITH EGER, Holocaust survivor, bestselling author, and esteemed lecturer

"Heather Chauvin is a truth-teller, and this book is a must-read for everyone. Heather's story will inspire you to release all unnecessary suffering and claim your magical life."

CATHY HELLER, author of *Don't Keep Your Day Job*

"Heather Chauvin's wisdom seeps through each story and lesson. The permission she offers mothers to let go and embrace their current selves as enough is a gift every mother needs upon rising each day. This book is for any mother who needs a gentle yet powerful reminder that your first priority is *you*— not motherhood, not marriage, just *you*."

SARA DEAN, host of *The Shameless Mom Academy* podcast

"Heather Chauvin writes with such refreshing honesty, painting a beautiful picture with her words in a way that makes you feel seen and understood. This book is a must-read for moms. I don't say that lightly... every mom should have access to these words."

ALLIE CASAZZA, host of *The Purpose* ~~~~~~~~~~~~~~ author of *Declutter Like a Mother*

D1115746

**Dying
to Be a
Good
Mother**

How I dropped the guilt and took control of my parenting and my life

HEATHER CHAUVIN

Dying to Be a Good Mother

PAGE TWO BOOKS

Cataloguing in publication information is available
from Library and Archives Canada.
ISBN 978-1-77458-022-6 (paperback)
ISBN 978-1-77458-023-3 (ebook)

Page Two
pagetwo.com

Edited by Emily Schultz
Copyedited by Rachel Ironstone
Proofread by Alison Strobel
Cover design by Corey Futko and Fiona Lee
Cover photo by Vicki Bartel
Interior design by Fiona Lee

heatherchauvin.com
dyingtobeagoodmother.com

To my grandmother, whose story was left unwritten,

and who gave me the courage to write mine.

Contents

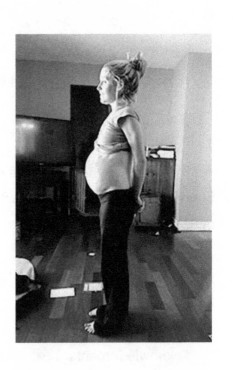

Introduction

'**M SMILING, OR** at least I'm trying to.

That's my first thought every time I see this photo. It was taken in December 2013. I was a twenty-seven-year-old married mom of three with a degree in social work. An increasingly devoted personal development junkie, I meditated, drank green juice, and was slowly growing my business helping moms take control of their lives. Honestly, though, it was proving to be an expensive, time-consuming hobby. We were under tremendous financial strain that was wearing badly on my marriage.

At first glance my smile seems appropriate, even heartwarming. The thing is, I wasn't pregnant; I had just been diagnosed with stage four cancer, specifically, Burkitt's lymphoma. My big belly? That held the rapidly growing abdominal tumors that doctors, nurses, and countless others assumed would kill me years before my youngest, then just one year old, would start school. This photo? That's me, faking a smile for the camera, knowing that I was at the *you're-totally-screwed* stage. (When you're potentially at death's door, about to shave your hair and spend the next several months with your head in a toilet bowl, keeping up appearances is everything... ha!)

Looking back, I could of course say that cancer changed my life; but that's only partly true. Cancer, for me, was a giant boot, a gargantuan steel toe, kicking me where it hurt most, forcing me to see what I already knew to be true.

My way of existing wasn't allowing me to exist. It was killing me—quickly and far too young.

After becoming a single mom at eighteen, I'd spent my young adult life trying—and as it turned out, literally dying—to be a good mother. Every feeling I experienced, every thought I had, every action I took was from a place of never being enough. No matter how depleted I felt, every day was about doing more, being more, giving more to everyone but myself. Motherhood was about self-sacrifice—well, that's what society told me, anyway.

I wish I could say I was the only one. I wish I could say that I don't still work with women who are living from this soul-sucking place of "never enough." Unfortunately, Western culture not only validates this impossible ideal around motherhood, offering quick-fix solutions like "wine o'clock" and extra caffeine, it also often judges women harshly for not self-sacrificing *enough*.

When my cancer diagnosis arrived, I had to step back and take a deeper look at motherhood, and what it meant to me. Up until that point, I'd bought into the idea that motherhood requires self-sacrifice; that no matter how much I did or gave, it would never truly be enough. After being diagnosed, I had to figure out how to let enough *feel* like enough. I had to stop dying to be a good mother and start *living* to be one.

It all sounds so simple, at first. *Just think differently! Make different choices!* I can do that. You can do that. No big deal... or is it?

As I write this, it's 2020, and I'm six years into being cancer-free. That girl in the photo? Sometimes I call her Old Heather.

I hardly recognize myself, or my life, for that matter. I'm healthier and happier than I have ever been. I've also built a thriving career guiding overwhelmed moms in becoming the authentic, heart-centered leaders that they were meant to be in their homes and throughout their lives. My relationships with my husband and three sons are never perfect, yet they all feel more nourishing and authentic.

Is it a miracle? Yes, absolutely, but it also required a lot of effort and dedication.

Before cancer, so much of what I did was for others. I began practicing meditation to help my firstborn manage *his* emotions. I taught mindfulness to help *other people's* kids. I helped friends and family navigate *their* challenges. I supported *other* overwhelmed moms in taking better care of *them*selves. I stood up when others fell down. I was the strong one. Do you ever feel like that woman—the one everyone needs? The fact is, feeling needed can feel good. However, placing so much focus on others also became the perfect excuse to neglect my own emotions, and the vulnerability they brought to the forefront. As long as I stayed busy playing the role of the rescuer, saving everyone who needed me, it was easier to avoid the one person I was terrified of rescuing—myself.

As I navigated chemotherapy and the months of recovery that followed, I had to stop avoiding the pain I'd tried so hard to stuff down. During the years since, I've had to take an honest look at my past, present, and future; at how I was talking to myself and, by extension, my kids, husband, family, and friends. Over and over again, I've had to find new ways of seeing, being, believing, and loving; of working, eating, exercising, and caring for my heart and soul. Finally, it all became so clear.

Heather, to continue nurturing others, you first have to nurture yourself.

Heather, to feel joy, you first have to be willing to receive love and support.

Heather, it's time to be you—the real you.

It all seems so obvious now, but as I coach the strong, bold, amazing women who gravitate toward me, I realize we're all in this together. At the end of the day, we're all dying to be ourselves—our imperfect, loving, and never-simple-but-rarely-boring selves.

Wherever you are in your journey, one thing I now know is that the little whisper inside you, that yearning to be the real you, the all-of-you you—is *so* important. That little voice inside you that's craving more joy, more fulfillment, more connection? It really might save your life.

And what we forget too often and too easily is that we have the one and only thing anyone ever needs.

We have time.

I don't often talk about this, but the truth is, I don't know why I'm still here. I don't know why I still *get* to be here, when so many beautiful, inspiring, giving, loving souls have left. Why me? Why not them? Why not all of us?

So many of us are waking up each day anticipating next month or next season, the start of the school year or the end of it. *That's* when we'll take action. *That's* when we'll make the change that we know we need to make. *That's* when we'll have the time and energy to listen to our heart's desires. What we're overlooking is that now, right now, is the greatest gift of all.

We're here. We *get* to be here. That's *everything*.

So many of us are running through our days, fake smiling through our heartaches, our soul aches, our life breakdowns. What cancer taught me is that suffering is not living. It's a form of dying—if not in body, then in heart and soul.

I'm writing this book because you can choose a new way. You can decide to really live, to nurture yourself alongside those you love and cherish. I want you to take a stand for yourself, and your dreams—and by extension, your children and who they're becoming as well.

In Part I, I share my personal journey, beginning with the unplanned blessing that arrived just eight weeks before my nineteenth birthday—my firstborn, Logan. He was my first greatest gift, my first Big Why for seeking a new path, a different way of living, loving, and thriving. Those shifts would unfold gradually, though. During my early years as a single mother, trying to get myself through university and then into a career, I struggled. Profoundly unprepared for motherhood, I fumbled my way through, always terrified that I was "ruining" my child—by being me, or by not being me. Good was never, ever good enough.

In Part II, I continue my journey, including my cancer diagnosis, treatment, and recovery. It was a shock, suddenly being torn from my home, my family, my life. Having to focus so much of my energy and attention on surviving, I had plenty of time to think. What came to light during this time changed me forever, drawing me deeper into the personal development journey that saved me in many critical ways.

To nudge you forward on your own personal journey, starting in this section I share a simple but powerful reflective exercise at the end of some chapters. I hope you take the time to complete these, ideally in a notebook or journal where you can record your thoughts and refer back to them later. You may be tempted to resist this, but trust me, it's going to be a game changer. Why wait for permission? You already have it. Together these exercises will help you get closer to the raw and real, true and beautiful you that may be spending far too much time hiding behind a brave and loving, but still fake-smiling, exterior.

In Part III, I continue my journey, fast-forwarding to the present and reflecting backward, as well as forward, on the challenges I have overcome, and those I still wrestle with. I also tell the stories of some of the amazing women I now coach. These incredible women are slowly but surely finding the courage to be the vibrant, strong, joyful leaders we were all meant to be. Using techniques that have helped me and them, I continue to provide a simple soul-seeking reflection at the end of each chapter.

As women, we do so much and give so much. We love so completely and nurture so many. Few embodied that as fully as my dear friends, Alison and Michelle. If there were a Nobel Prize for spirit, they would have won it. This book is also for them, and every mother like them, who lived each moment to the fullest, giving to everyone around them with their whole heart. To the very end they fought with a courage and a tenacity that should inspire us all to use each moment we get to really live and really love, not just for others but for ourselves also.

Your perfect time to start? It's now. It's *right now*. Tomorrow, next week, next month—it won't feel easier. I know you have lots of laundry to finish, I know your to-do list is endless, and I know you're thinking, *I don't have time to read this book*. But when are you going to stop using motherhood as the excuse to not take care of yourself? Trust me, it gets easier, but you have to give yourself permission to create space for what you truly want. Take five minutes, read a few words, and know you're not alone. When we show up for this journey, we can make magic happen. Come and join me—let's dive in together, because together we can do almost anything.

Heather

PART I

Dying to Be a Good Mother

1

Embracing the Good

PEOPLE OFTEN ASK ME how I can smile and laugh when I say I had stage four cancer. I usually respond that it's either because I'm in complete denial—which I don't believe is the case, but no one's perfect, so I won't rule it out—or because I've healed that part of myself.

As this chapter is being written, it's April 2020, my sixth anniversary of being cancer-free. It's a milestone I once wasn't sure I'd see, and one that I can't entirely explain. Looking back, however, some things are clear. First, the personal development work I have done, and continue to do, has saved my life and transformed it in the process. Also, and perhaps most important, motherhood, which I often call "personal growth on steroids," is a powerful and unyielding mirror, a sacred invitation into ourselves, and our best life—if and when we choose to accept it.

Cancer did save my life, but it's only one part of my story. What cancer also did is show me that I am worthy of feeling alive and living a full life. Actually learning how to *feel* alive and then figuring out how to live that way were lessons I had to very intentionally seek out post-recovery. It was a journey—it still is one—and one of the most profoundly challenging and rewarding experiences of my life.

Ultimately, though, what I've realized is that these lessons aren't really about me. They're about all of us, as women, and our desire and struggle to break free from the limitations that we take on in order to embody others' definition of what we should be—a "good" mother and "good" wife and "good" daughter and so on. Far too often, we spend our days caring for everyone else and rarely take time or energy to care for ourselves. This commitment to self-sacrifice, I eventually realized, was why I nearly died trying to be a "good" mother.

Now, all these years later, I see how doing the work to show up as myself and for myself, as well as the thousands of mothers I coach, has allowed me to become healthier than I've ever been. While my health is in part a reflection of the habits I try to adhere to—nourishing my body with wholesome foods, moving my body regularly, doing the emotional and spiritual work, and embracing my ongoing commitment to feeling better than I did yesterday—my abundant energy and well-being are also reflections of how I'm showing up as a mother, coach, and leader.

Like most women, I still struggle with challenging emotions like fear and guilt, but I also see them as energies I can co-create with. Waiting for the day when we're not afraid or feeling any guilt is unrealistic; more often than not, it's an excuse to avoid facing ourselves and the goals and desires we've abandoned.

Partly because I no longer resist challenging emotions, I've become the authentic, visionary leader I long dreamed of being. Women sometimes tell me that I appear confident and bold—and I am both of those things, but I also often experience intense anxiety. Even now, I still feel uneasy when I send a new email out to my list. Rarely does a week go by that I don't fear that I will lose all of my clients because I've said the "wrong" thing. While I can be very outspoken, I am also very sensitive. It's beautiful feeling so connected, but it's also intensely draining. In spite of all of these contradictions and complexities—and maybe even because of them—I have never felt as alive, energized, and abundant as I now feel most days.

Since my early (pre-cancer) years of hustling in my business, I have realized that working endlessly—and being reactionary rather than focused and proactive—comes from a place of fear and lack. It's also a pattern that's been passed down through the patriarchy. This may seem ironic, but it was only when cancer forced me to stop overworking that I was able to achieve the level of success and abundance I desired. Working with a powerful and committed team has made all the difference, allowing me to serve more clients at a higher level.

I love my work and feel deeply committed to my clients, but I no longer use work as an excuse to deny or ignore my own needs and desires. Instead, I see work as one way to fulfill my purpose and make a bigger impact on the world, but never in a self-sacrificing way.

One of cancer's many other gifts was showing me the power of community. In the years since my diagnosis, getting groups of like-minded women together, both online and in person (when that's possible), is a deeply transformative act of healing, and one that I use in my work and my life often. When we, as women, come together and commit to embodying our best selves, positivity and potential become almost contagious, transforming us and our lives in amazing ways.

Like most women, I'm not immune to feelings of unworthiness, but since cancer, I've also stayed committed to thriving rather than surviving. Now, I constantly ask myself, *How good can my life get?* It's a big and sometimes scary question for someone with dreams like mine, but also an important one that I encourage clients to ask themselves too. How good can your life get? What about your best friend's? Your mother's? Your daughter's?

Every week, I help women answer that question by guiding them toward ways to regain control over their lives and achieve emotional freedom, which is the ability to feel and move through the emotions that have been holding them captive. Invariably, the process includes looking at parenting challenges in entirely new ways. The fact is, we can't understand our children when we don't fully understand and accept ourselves. More often than not, addressing parenting issues involves looking at yourself first and foremost. This means finally embracing the idea that self-care and feeling good are the opposite of selfish; that we can't show up for others if we're not first showing up for ourselves.

The simple fact I now know and live by is that when I feel good and show up as my best self, I radiate positive energy that allows other women to do the same for themselves, in their lives. At the end of the day, we can either trigger or inspire the people we surround ourselves with. I aim to inspire women, and to show them that they, too, are worthy of more.

But getting to this place has been an extended process of self-discovery that began early and in the most unexpected of ways.

2

This Changes Everything

"**M**OM."

She waved her hand, brushing me off.

"*Mom*," I repeated, this time a little louder.

I could feel my gut swirling as fear, dread, and shame began brewing inside me. A few more agonizing seconds passed. This was real. This was happening. I couldn't wait any longer.

"What's wrong with you?" she asked, irritated to see that my face had become a puddle of tears.

You're a bother, Heather. You don't matter this much. They were thoughts I'd heard echo inside me many times before. This was different though. This time I needed her.

"Can you get off the phone? I need to talk to you."

Fed up with the intense cramps I'd been having, I'd taken a pregnancy test from the health clinic where I worked part-time, after school. Expecting a negative result, and figuring I had a urinary tract infection, I'd squatted over the toilet and peed into a shot glass I'd taken from my mom's cabinet. Two lines had appeared immediately. Paralyzed by shock and fear, I'd collapsed on the floor and wept. Moments later, here I was trying to get my mom's attention.

"Mom," I repeated, my voice jagged and edgy.

Finally, she ended her call.

Speak, Heather. You have to say the words now. I swallowed, my heart thumping in my chest. It was time to fess up to being the fuck-up everyone knew I'd become.

"Mom," I began, dying to get this moment over with, but also wishing I could delay, maybe change things somehow, rewind the clock and put this off, at least for a few years. "I'm pregnant."

She stared back at me, her face blank, yet dark too.

"Oh my God. Oh my God. Oh my God."

Was she going to scream? Give me shit? Disown me? My panic mounting, I stood facing her, tears cascading down my cheeks. I craved comfort, affection, reassurance. I wanted, needed, to feel less alone, less terrified, more of anything that might make me feel even a tiny bit calmer, steadier, safer in my body, my life.

"Oh my God. Oh my God. Oh my God."

She stood still, repeating those words for what seemed like thirty minutes. Then, with hardly another word, she gathered her things and left to go to my uncle's house. He had always been her go-to, the one person she talked to when she needed advice and support.

Alone in her house, the contrast was painfully clear: She had someone who cared for her and supported her. I had no one. *You're not good enough, Heather. You'll never be that important.* My self-talk reverberated inside me, rocking me to my core, not because it was new or different, but because this time I had proof. Those two lines were confirmation of what I'd always feared—that I was going to amount to absolutely nothing in my life.

Also, I was pregnant with *his* baby. Not yet ready to face that fact, or what it could mean for me and my child, I tried to push that thought away. It was only three weeks until graduation. I could hide my middle until then. No one at school would have to know. That, at least, provided some relief.

Looking back, though, my real secret wasn't that I'd gotten pregnant. It was something I wouldn't admit to myself, or anyone else, for years to come. On some level I hadn't consciously acknowledged yet, I had wanted this. A baby, *my* baby, would love me. As a mother, I would finally feel loved and, most of all, worthy of love.

Now that it was happening, though, it all felt so different. I had wanted this, sure, but never as a teen, and definitely not by him. This was too soon. I was only eighteen years old. I had no money, and, yet again, I'd be left alone to clean up my mess.

You're going to be a statistic, Heather. You're the fucking failure everyone knew you'd become.

After years of managing undiagnosed depression and suicidal thoughts, never feeling good enough at school, college was finally in sight. For me college was about more than getting a degree. It was my way out. It was how I would finally escape from the small town I'd grown up in. It was how I'd travel the world and discover a new life, *my* life. But now that I was on the verge of becoming a single teen mom, what would happen to me? Would I even make it to college?

Soon after telling my mom the news, I returned to the clinic and confessed to Dr. Patterson, who did rounds there, that I might be pregnant. He nodded, led me into an exam room, and proceeded to do an ultrasound. I was shocked to discover that I was already twelve weeks. Looking back, it's hard to believe that I was that disconnected from my body. Nearly into my second trimester, I hadn't even taken notice of all of the ways that it had been changing.

As Dr. Patterson completed his exam, I looked over at him. "Thank you, Dr. Patterson."

He looked at me, surprised and a little confused.

"For not judging me," I added.

He nodded and shrugged, unfazed. *This is my job*, he seemed to be communicating, as if judging me, a pregnant single teen, hadn't occurred to him. After I confessed to having mixed feelings about this pregnancy, he suggested that I go see his wife, a therapist. I gladly took her card. I'd been to therapy a few times before and loved it. To me it was an opportunity to learn more about psychology and the brain, a topic that, even then, never failed to capture my attention.

Scraping together the money to pay Dr. Judy wasn't easy—at eighty dollars per session, she was way above my budget—but I did it anyway. During our brief time together—I went to see her a few times, until it was clear I couldn't afford her anymore—she listened to me and explained what anxiety was. It was the first time I'd heard the word, and the first time I'd been able to name the emotional dis-ease I'd long felt. (Just five years later, my son, by then in elementary school, would begin learning how to use meditation to manage anxiety, and here I was, eighteen years old, hearing the word for the very first time.)

MISSING MOST of the first trimester of my pregnancy could have made the remaining two trimesters fly by. Instead, the days, weeks, and months dragged out into an endless, miserable blur. Throughout, I felt fat, bloated, and depleted. While most of my friends spent their post-graduation months drinking and celebrating, I spent much of my time napping. Sleep, I realized years later, was my coping strategy. It was my drug of choice, how I numbed out and avoided living my life.

As lonely as I was, being at home with my mom wasn't any easier. Throughout my pregnancy, we co-existed in her house but barely spoke to one another. She'd made it clear that I was no longer welcome, but since I didn't yet have any other place to go, I stayed. While she dealt with her own complicated emotions around my situation, I felt isolated and disowned, like a blemish everyone wished would go away. My dad, who wasn't thrilled about my pregnancy either, had reluctantly offered me a place to live. While I appreciated the gesture, I never seriously considered his offer. He'd remarried when I was two years old, and I'd only ever lived with him for short periods of time. Even in my desperate situation, moving into his house with an infant didn't seem like a realistic option.

My dad and stepmom showed their support in other ways, too, extending my job at the campground my dad owned beyond the usual peak summer season. Through the fall and into the early winter months, they continued to pay me well for the low-level work I was doing, often throwing in gas money and groceries. Their support was consistent, but their message was clear—they would continue to employ me, as long as I was willing to work. As fall turned into winter, I spent long hours completing inventory and getting the campground ready for springtime. It wasn't exciting work, but it was available, and I needed every dollar I could earn.

As my due date neared, I felt more depressed than ever, but still, I clung to my dream of going to college, if not university. I wasn't at all sure that either would be possible, but I knew that I couldn't keep doing what I was doing. I would soon have an infant to care for. I would need a reliable source of income.

Committed to doing what was best for my baby, I stood in line with a friend one day to apply for the Canadian equivalent of welfare. I felt ashamed and scared that I really was becoming a teen mom statistic, but there would be another mouth to feed, and the clock was ticking. The application process proved longer and more difficult than I expected. Weeks of paperwork followed me, and throughout, I searched frantically for housing. I was fine with living alone, but continually disappointed by the high cost of housing. Where would I live? How would I support myself and my baby? My growing belly was a constant reminder of the overwhelming uncertainty surrounding me.

As weeks turned into months, my mom and I were still barely speaking. When I was seven or eight months pregnant, at the recommendation of my uncle, she and I went to see a relationship counselor. The therapist was a blunt, bold woman, and I felt an immediate kinship with her. During that session, she took a stand for me by acknowledging and validating my emotions. Not long afterward, my mom allowed me to move into her basement, which is what I'd wanted to do, since the basement was more spacious than my upstairs bedroom. The atmosphere in the house was still tense, but finally, I had a place to live once the baby arrived.

ON JANUARY 11, 2005, I went into the hospital to give birth. Past my due date by that point, my doctor had recommended that I be induced. When I arrived at my scheduled check-in time, some of my stepmom's friends, who were nurses at the hospital, sought me out and went out of their way to make me as comfortable as possible. I was grateful, but incredibly overwhelmed, and deeply unnerved by the possibility of my ex-boyfriend, the baby's father, coming to the hospital for the birth.

We'd stayed in touch throughout my pregnancy; he'd called almost weekly to check in. I hated hearing from him, but usually made myself pick up the call, since this was, after all, his baby too.

Who was he? Do you remember that disarmingly charming disaster you fell head over heels for in high school? Mine was named John. We'd met the year before in night school, which

I'd had to attend due to poor grades. He was four years older than me and suffered from drug addiction and mental health issues. However, I was a high school girl, and he was good-looking and also attentive when we were together. By the time I noticed that he was always high and continually swapped out coffee for beer, I was already lost in those beautiful eyes of his.

Fairly soon after settling into my hospital bed on that bitter cold January day, it became clear that the birth wouldn't be any easier than the pregnancy had been. I felt overwhelmed by all of the people there, which included my mom and several other friends and relatives. Eventually, John, his mom, and stepdad, Mark, also arrived. It wasn't at all what I'd expected. My room felt like a fucking circus. I was the main attraction, the tiger, terrified of catching on fire as I jumped through the hoop, all eyes fixed on me.

To get the birth process started, the doctors gave me Pitocin, which is standard protocol. Things progressed, but slowly. I remember being on all fours, my legs splayed open and my ass hanging out, screaming from the intense pain of contractions, feeling exposed and humiliated.

At one point a mass of nurses and doctors rushed into the room announcing that the baby was in distress. Paperwork was shoved in front of me as medical staff gathered around my bed, telling me to sign, and if I didn't, my baby would die. To this day I have no idea why they bother having you sign those papers. By that point, you're completely traumatized, and there's no way you can make sense of the specific legal clauses you're agreeing to. If ever there were a case for pleading temporary insanity, or at least a profound inability to think logically, labor is it.

Terrified, and not at all clear about what I was agreeing to, or what rights I was signing away, I did what any mother would do and signed every paper they shoved in front of me.

Consumed by the general sense of panic in the room, all I knew was that they were going to do a C-section, which I'd never wanted. I remember saying, "No, not this. No, I didn't want it to happen like this," as they wheeled me toward the operating room.

As soon as we got into the OR, I begged the doctor not to let John into the room, unsure what he might do if he went into one of his delusions, which came on suddenly and were often scary. Since they had to either let everyone in or no one, they closed the room off to all visitors. I briefly worried that my mom's feelings would be hurt, but knew she'd understand that I wanted to protect the baby from John. Moments later, as I lay on the operating table, I asked the surgeon if he was cutting my belly. Realizing that the epidural they'd given me earlier had worn off, a nurse immediately lowered a mask onto my face.

Oh my God, this is real. I'm a mother now.

I'd been unconscious for the entire birth, so having a baby in my arms felt odd, shocking even. As I looked down at his beautiful, bubbly little face, I felt a fierce, bold energy coursing through my body. In that split second, I became his mama bear. *I've got you. I'm going to protect you. I'm going to show up for you.* More than any other, that moment and that promise I made to my son changed my life forever. I had a mission now, a legacy to uphold. If I couldn't show up for myself, I would show up for this precious baby boy in my arms. Logan.

As everyone oohed and aahed, Logan was passed around to friends and relatives. At one point, when John walked into the room holding him, my heart leapt from fear of what he might do. Thankfully, in that moment he was being sweet-and-charming John, paying loving attention to our newly born baby.

I lay there as family and friends took pictures and talked beyond the curtain that surrounded my bed. Still traumatized by the birth, I was too sore and too overwhelmed to move or participate in the conversation. I felt isolated and detached, almost like an invisible presence everyone knew was there, but no one acknowledged.

After passing Logan to another family member, John came through the curtain, sat down on the bed, and pulled out a knife.

"Heather," he began. "This baby should not be alive."

I wasn't yet in college, but already I felt drawn to social work. I'd had no formal training, but somehow, I knew how to deescalate the situation.

"What do you mean?" I asked, feeling my fear while trying to look and sound even-keeled, almost nonchalant.

"There are spies all around," he continued, explaining that other people would hurt Logan. I remember thinking, *He's going to harm Logan in an attempt to protect him.* When John got up, I looked over at John's stepdad.

"Mark," I said, smiling. "Can you please get security?"

Mark and I got along, mostly because we agreed about the seriousness of John's mental health issues. As soon I spoke, he nodded, immediately understanding what was happening. I calmly asked a friend to bring Logan to me. John soon picked up on what was happening, but by then security had arrived. They quickly escorted him out, his arms held behind his back. John's parting words to me were, "You will not take my son away from me."

Just watch me, I remember thinking as I held onto my little boy. Not long after, I was moved to a new hospital room and given the authority to approve every visitor before they were permitted to enter that room.

Three days later, I went home to my mom's basement. A new mother, a brave and fierce mama bear, I was terrified that John would reappear when and where I least expected. Desperate for support and protection, I begged the boy I had dated for years in high school, prior to John, to stay with me at my mom's house. His presence was a gift. Thanks to him, for that first week or two, I was able to rest and care for Logan without worrying that we were in danger.

AFTER SEVERAL extended delays, my government checks began to arrive. Literally overnight, I had a steady income that was higher than anything I'd ever earned. Being able to support myself and Logan provided welcome relief, but it also made me uncomfortable. My mom and I had lived in a trailer park for years, but she and everyone in my family had worked hard to support themselves. Up until this point, going on welfare hadn't been part of my world. It wasn't something people in my family did, yet here I was, cashing every government check that arrived.

Still terrified of becoming a single teen mom statistic, I immediately began looking forward. *What happens when these checks stop coming? How will I support us then?* Fighting exhaustion and with no alternate childcare, I decided that I had two options. I could either get a part-time job, earn less than I was getting from the government, and hate my life forever. Or, I could use these benefits to support me and Logan while I went to school and pursued a degree.

At the time my decision seemed like a no-brainer, but it could have easily felt harder than it did. After all, I was still chronically depressed and felt very lonely. I also frequently suffered from headaches, and sometimes nausea and vomiting too. On every level—physical, mental, and emotional—the idea of buckling down to apply for benefits and then studying to get a degree was beyond overwhelming. Something had shifted in me, though. Going back to school wasn't about me anymore. I was taking a stand for Logan's future, and to do that, I first had to take a stand for my own.

As I got further into the process of applying for benefits and then for school, some of the choices I'd made in high school came back to haunt me. My grades were poor, mostly due to lack of effort. I'd also chosen to take fewer academic classes, figuring I wasn't good enough for university. As a result, in order to qualify for college or university, I'd first have to complete a general year to take the required classes that I was missing. It would also be my chance to prove to the government system that was funding my life that I was serious about school this time.

It was a setback, sure, but not something I would let stop me. When Logan was eight months old, I enrolled him in the best childcare I could afford and resumed a full-time student schedule. Throughout that preliminary year, I studied consistently and did well. Every step of the way, Logan was my squirmy, noise-making little study buddy, and I sometimes brought him to class with me instead of dropping him off at daycare. He was my world, my life, my one and only reason for trying.

As that academic year progressed and he began turning into a toddler, I faced another choice. I could either apply to become a child and youth worker, which would mean completing a three-year college program. Or, I could apply to university and get a social work degree, which meant a four-year program but would qualify me for better jobs down the line.

One extra year of school was all it would take to get the degree I wanted but had always assumed would be out of my reach. I remember thinking, *If I can have a baby at eighteen, I can get a university degree*. With Logan in tow, for the first time I didn't care what other people thought I could or couldn't do. I didn't ask anyone's permission to apply to university and didn't care when people told me what I was doing would be too hard or take too long. I was a mother now. This wasn't about me.

After getting accepted to the four-year university program I wanted, I took out a loan to pay for it. I also continued to pursue every government benefit I qualified for. Being able to collect welfare during summer breaks allowed me to spend that time with Logan. I also got periodic stipends, like a warm clothing check in winter, and knew I could get extra money for diapers if I ever needed it.

As time passed, I began to see how government support could act almost like a drug, making life so much easier. While I appreciated having that sense of security, I still carried a lot of guilt about receiving government assistance. Ultimately, though, my commitment to Logan, and our future, prevented me from stopping short of earning my degree. Those government checks were how I was getting us to a better life, a self-supporting life. I needed them, I continued to remind myself, but only for now.

While my grades remained good, my poor health continued to drain my energy. Still sleeping as much as I could, I dealt with my perpetual exhaustion by staying busy. Although I had minimal energy, if I had to get to class, or go pick up Logan or study or be somewhere, I could keep going. Looking back, that should have been a clue, a sign that my exhaustion wasn't a physical need. It was the dark cloud of depression that had been hovering over me since childhood. I didn't need more sleep. I needed hope. I needed inspiration, love, and nurturing. Instead, I continued to focus on doing more and giving more to everyone but myself.

Wanting to give Logan the sense of family I hadn't always felt—my parents had divorced when I was very young—one Thanksgiving, I decided I would cook the annual family feast. It felt like what I was supposed to do, both as a mother and as a woman. Making that meal was an especially big leap for me, since eating had long been something I blew off, as if my body was somehow devoid of the basic human need for food and water. Most days I relied on coffee for energy, barely bothering to eat at all. The kitchen, for me at that time, was where I went to feed Logan.

Making multiple recipes on that Thanksgiving Day felt hard and unnatural, like a lot of bother for one silly meal. Yet again, though, this was for Logan. He would feel the love, warmth, and connection of family, even if I hadn't. Hours later, once I'd finished cooking, I felt so depleted that I lay down and napped for several hours. I remember blaming the time I'd spent on my feet for my exhaustion, but I was in my early twenties at the time, far too young for standing to tire me out. Unable to shake my exhaustion from one day to the next, I would occasionally complain to someone about my perpetual fatigue. Almost without fail, I'd get the same response. "You have a young one. You're a mom now. That's normal." It felt like validation for my long-standing habit of pushing my health aside.

By the time I was approaching the end of my university studies, I had more than a degree and career ahead of me. My personal life, too, had changed dramatically. When Logan was eighteen months old, right before I'd begun university, I'd attended a friend's wedding and met a guy named Bryan. Not yet ready to trust men, I did everything in my power to push him away.

"Logan is my top priority."

"I don't have time for you."

"I have to study."

"I'm done with men."

My excuses for not seeing Bryan were numerous, but ultimately, they proved ineffective. He genuinely loves kids and quickly bonded with Logan. Eventually, I relaxed and realized that I didn't want to shake him. Our relationship progressed naturally, and when Logan was three years old, we moved out of my mom's basement and into Bryan's house.

From the outside, my life and Logan's life at Bryan's house looked normal and steady. For at least that first year living together, though, I felt like a couch surfer with her young son in tow. Bryan rejected that idea completely, reassuring me that we were a unit. I couldn't yet go there, though. Still super protective of Logan, I wasn't yet willing to get that comfortable or trust that deeply.

Early in my fourth year of university, I'd gotten pregnant. Due in late November 2009, just weeks before my university graduation, I anticipated transitioning into a social work career, and becoming mom to a second child, with my usual resigned determination. Still spending as many of my waking hours with Logan as I could, I studied and focused on graduating.

As I neared the last trimester of my pregnancy, I was scheduled to begin my last semester of university, and Logan was to start kindergarten. But just my luck, that September saw the beginning of a massive university-wide strike, which resulted in weeks of canceled classes. With Logan in school and my classes temporarily suspended, I was faced with a void that I hadn't seen coming. With nowhere to go, and no Logan to go there with, I felt hollow and purposeless. Once again, I returned to my bed, sleeping my days away, awakening each afternoon just before Logan got home from school. After weeks of this, I got so depressed, I spent an entire week painting and repainting our living room, eventually settling on a depressing shade of shit brown. Finally, the strike ended. Relieved, I resumed a full-time university student schedule. In October 2009, a couple of months before I was scheduled to complete my university studies, not long before our baby was due, Bryan and I married. My cousin and her boyfriend looked on as witnesses.

I'M PRETTY SURE there's no love at first sight quite like holding your newborn in your arms for the very first time. It's such a big love, an all-consuming love, that you doubt you'll feel it quite like that ever again.

Throughout my second pregnancy, like many women, I worried that I wouldn't be able to love my second child as much as I loved Logan. What we forget in that place of fear and anxiety is that our capacity to love is limitless; that as mothers, loving our children is one of our superpowers. As our family grows, so, too, does our capacity to love and nurture.

When they placed Calvin in my arms, my heart exploded once again. He was beautiful. He was perfect. He was ours. At long last, I could see how much of our life had changed. Logan had Bryan and now a baby brother, too, whom he loved and bonded with almost immediately. We were a family now. Finally, I let myself feel it, and what had been Bryan's house gradually began to feel like our home. A piece of me could finally relax, trust, and breathe a huge sigh of relief.

During Calvin's first few weeks at home, as he adjusted to life outside of the womb, I completed my university projects, taking a break from my field assignments that spring to spend more time with him. The following summer, when Calvin was about six months old, I completed my final university requirements and earned my degree. The different field placements I completed during those months working with high-risk families and people experiencing homelessness proved to be life-changing experiences that shaped me and my social work career for years to come. During those years, I discovered the true depth of motherhood and the distance a mother will go for her child. I also saw how we are all one, and that we need to come together as women instead of judging and breaking each other down.

3

Dying to Be a
Good Mother Syndrome

WHY HAS MATERNAL EXHAUSTION become a badge of honor? How has it become socially acceptable, even admirable, to give so much that your body and soul are prematurely dying from lack of rest and spiritual replenishment?

This feels like a new cultural trend, but is it, really? My mother and her mother and her mother's mother all believed that they didn't matter. Why is that? Why is being a mother openly viewed as one of the most undervalued positions we can have, yet so much of human development is attached to the health and well-being of the mother?

We see and define motherhood in ways that are contradictory and self-defeating. Once I became a mother of two, my life began to reflect those deeply held cultural beliefs around motherhood to an even greater degree. Eventually, I began to refer to it as the Dying to Be a Good Mother syndrome.

Absorbing the Shock

Calvin's abundant energy might have been some sort of cosmic correction. Almost from the moment he exited my womb, he was in constant motion. Maybe the Universe was having a laugh on me, or just putting its sense of humor on display. Whatever the case, Calvin's boundless energy, and the ongoing demands it created, was a huge shock to my system.

During the last months of my pregnancy with Calvin, who was born in December, I'd slept and slept. That September, as I was heading into my final trimester of my pregnancy, Logan had begun junior kindergarten (JK), which is Canada's rough equivalent of kindergarten. His weekday absence felt raw and wrong, like a special kind of torture designed just for me. I agonized often, worrying how he felt in school and whether he was making friends, what he was eating and whether he was safe. Most of all, though, I struggled with larger-than-life guilt. Was I a "good" mother? Was I doing enough? Was I doing enough of the "right" things? I measured my every move against some unwritten rule book, grasping for confidence but always finding more reasons to doubt myself.

Eager for guidance and direction, over the years I'd attended some moms' groups but had left each one keenly aware of the gaps in age and life experiences. I was, as a rule, the only mom in those groups who'd had her first child at age eighteen. Unlike my own, the lives of the moms in those groups looked impossibly perfect and shiny, or so I thought at the time. Unwilling to subject myself to more judgment, I resorted to soaking up whatever information I could. At school functions, in coffee shops, at work, and out with Logan, I watched, listened, and learned. What were other moms doing? What were *they* focusing on? As I absorbed tips and tidbits from other moms around me, I made one mental note after another about what I needed to do and stop doing, do more of and not do at all. Each new piece of information felt useful, but also highlighted the distance between the "good" moms and me.

At one point, I'd heard other moms of JK kids talk about wanting to follow the school bus, insisting that they had to be sure, with their own eyes, that their child arrived safely. Determined to measure up as a "good" mother, I announced one day that I'd be following behind the school bus in my car. Bryan looked at me like I'd lost my mind. I didn't need to, he insisted. Logan would be fine, he said, trying, but failing, to reassure me.

While Logan acclimated to JK, and the eggplant-sized being in my belly grew into the newborn we would soon meet, my only obligation was studying for final exams. I was scheduled to take them in December or, more likely, several months afterward, since Calvin was due to arrive at exam time. With my class requirements fulfilled, my schedule was suddenly, and rather overwhelmingly, blank. There was nowhere I had to be each day, nothing I absolutely had to accomplish on any given weekday.

Feeling off-kilter emotionally and physically uncomfortable from pregnancy, and with Bryan working long hours, I drifted through my days, alone and aimless. Every weekday, I'd wake up in time to get Logan ready for school, walk him to his bus stop, and then return home after his bus had driven safely away. Once back home, with nothing to do and nowhere I had to be, I'd lay down on the couch and sleep... and sleep. Waking up only to eat and meet Logan at the bus stop in the afternoons, I spent the bulk of my days in a hauntingly unsatisfying slumber—too anxious to sleep and too depressed not to.

Looking back, I can now see that being without Logan terrified me most because it was an in-my-face reminder that I had no real purpose without my child at my side. At the time, however, all I knew was that I desperately wanted to avoid feeling the deep pain I felt when Logan wasn't with me. Drifting in and out of sleep every Monday through Friday was unfulfilling but also less painful than being awake enough to look at myself and my life. Deep down, I was angry at Bryan for showing up as a parent for Logan (that had always been *my* job). I was also afraid that Logan wasn't being cared for at school the way I was sure he needed to be. Most of all, and for reasons I couldn't yet explain, I felt a deep and crushing sadness.

It was all too much for me to handle at that point in my life, so, as I'd done during my teenage years, I used sleep to numb out and avoid feeling my emotions. I could, and always did, rally when Logan was around me, but the rest of the time, I struggled with even the simplest of self-care tasks, including feeding myself, often opting to sleep instead.

The Picture of Success

At long last, Calvin arrived, and my heart—all of our hearts—leapt with joy. We were a family now, a foursome, not just in the house, but legally too. To protect Logan from his addict father, Bryan had adopted him, and now that I'd given birth to Calvin, Logan also had a baby brother. We were a unit and we were safe. It was a relief, knowing that we were creating a stable family life.

That feeling, however soothing, turned out to be more tenuous than I'd hoped. Months earlier, Bryan and I had bought a house. Still a full-time student at that point, I wasn't yet earning any money, and we knew my starting salary in social work would only slightly increase our household income. With Bryan working in the corporate world, there was no denying that he was, and would remain for the near future, the primary breadwinner.

When friends and family repeatedly referred to "Bryan's house," I of course knew what they meant. I got the fact that he'd supplied the down payment and was, for the moment, the only one paying the mortgage. I understood that many of those same people meant no real harm when they casually, even thoughtlessly, referred to our home as "Bryan's." Yet also, I couldn't shake the feeling that their words had a bigger, deeper meaning. We were married, preparing to welcome a child of our own, yet still, I was living in "his" house. Would Logan and I ever truly belong? Would I ever feel like anything more than a couch surfer?

It was a strangely contradictory existence, even after Calvin's arrival. On the one hand, we were legitimate—a real, true family of four. Still, though, I felt those old feelings—of playing the part of the married mom, yet never being quite enough; of not quite belonging with other moms or even in my own home. We looked legitimate, sure, but I still felt like the broken link in the chain.

Some months after Calvin's birth, soon after passing all of my university final exams, I landed a coveted, part-time job in social work. If ever there were a time to celebrate, this should have been it. I had, after all, *done it*. I'd defied the odds by getting a university degree. Now I had *the* job that so many in my graduating class had aspired to. Really, I should have been shouting from the rooftops, over the moon with pride and joy at having achieved the impossible as a young and previously poor, single mother. But of course, I didn't. I couldn't let myself feel, much less feel good. Even in the best of times, I needed to numb out and push away the many emotions I'd never be fully ready for.

Undeniably, though, from the outside, our life, and even I, *looked* successful. Now a mother of two with a "good" job, I was faced with a new and unknown challenge—raising a child with someone else. This wasn't my first rodeo as a mom, but for the first time my parenting decisions needed someone else's input. Never before had I had to integrate another adult's viewpoint on schedules, activities, playmates, and school. Being a family of four felt more legitimate, yes, but as I was learning, that legitimacy came with its challenges. In many ways I was starting over as a mom, having to figure out an entirely new way to parent, or, rather, co-parent. Now there was someone else to change a diaper. That might have felt like a blessing if I hadn't been so sure that self-sacrifice was the ultimate measure of my status as an aspiring "good" mother.

The "Curse" of Compassion

Starting my new job in social work did little to quiet my need to do everything possible for my two boys. Charged with observing visits with families that were being monitored by the government, I tried to maintain a safe emotional distance, but that didn't feel right. Many of the kids had suffered enormously and would be removed from their parents' homes. Witnessing these moments, and the pain that passed between them, was heartbreaking, emotionally draining work.

One of the reasons I'd been drawn to this position was because it came with part-time hours, which would give me more time with Logan and Calvin. While it did give me that, it also added pressure, since every moment I wasn't working, I felt I had to be with my boys. I gave myself no time to recover and little time to rest. My guilt about working, even part-time, felt heavy. The idea of taking even more time to take care of myself seemed downright selfish, even neglectful—the opposite of what any "good" mother would do.

At the same time, I couldn't ignore the growing evidence that I wasn't cut out for social work. The pain that the kids and their moms endured too easily became my pain—and something I had to "fix," which was also my way of avoiding my own unmet needs. Each of their stories would always make me want to get more emotionally involved, even when doing so wasn't in their best interest or mine. I simply couldn't detach emotionally from their suffering.

Every day I worked my social work shift, it also became clearer that I would never be able to create the kind of clear, definable impact I yearned to have. The size and complexity of the system required it to function in ways I didn't feel comfortable with. The system would always determine what was and wasn't possible, regardless of how it affected people's lives.

Wandering in a New Direction

Calvin was about six months old when I attended my first-ever retreat. It was a weekend-long event in Asheville, North Carolina, and the trip had been planned on what at the time seemed like a whim. After reading a book about children's meditation, I went online and noticed on the author's website that she would soon be hosting a retreat, educating those interested in teaching their children meditation. Following a gut instinct (and overlooking the fact that I couldn't afford to attend), I purchased a ticket.

The retreat was only a couple of flights away, but by the time I arrived, I felt like I'd traveled to a different world. We meditated and ate nourishing organic food, all the while surrounded by serene natural beauty. Spending that much time in meditation, I began to experience internal shifts that hinted at a whole new kind of healing. Fascinated by this new world and the potential it brought to light, I left Asheville amazed by the possibilities that meditation, and the entire health and wellness world, opened up. Yet at the same time, the mere idea of living like this—of meditating regularly and eating whole foods, for example—completely overwhelmed me. I could barely stick to a schedule, much less commit to a regular spiritual practice, and something as simple as cutting open an avocado sounded impossibly foreign to me.

While the health and wellness world felt intimidating, it also lit me up in ways I couldn't ignore. Soon after returning home, I began hosting kids' meditation classes at a retail space close to our house. Word began to spread, and the classes eventually moved to a yoga studio. Some also took place in my living room, where I occasionally taught while breastfeeding Calvin.

From the beginning, I charged a nominal fee for my classes, yet remained in total denial about the fact that I was planting the first seeds of a side business. I'd spent my entire life watching my dad work endless hours in his business and knew that I didn't want that schedule. Also, I was sure I didn't have "what it takes" to own a business. Yet at the same time, I knew that I had to do something to plan for the future. If social work wasn't a viable long-term option for me, I had to figure out what was.

Within a relatively short period of time, my days off from social work turned into a flurry of teaching, planning, and expanding whatever this thing I was building would become. Newly aware of the idea that our thoughts become things, I felt empowered to turn my new passion for health and wellness into something tangible.

Still racked with guilt about "never doing enough" as a mom, I spent all possible waking hours with my kids, playing, nursing, and feeding them before, after, and sometimes while working on my business. The idea of hiring a babysitter so I could work on my business or take some time for myself felt impossibly self-indulgent. I was, as they say, "doing it all," but also, I was exhausted and mentally, emotionally, and physically depleted. As always, though, I felt sure that I needed to give, give, and give more to my boys, as well as to my students, and even their moms. So I did the "right" thing and ignored my body's cries for attention.

As word of my classes began to spread, the groups began to grow. It was encouraging, but also complicated. Assuming that I was available simply because I was home, one mom got in the habit of dropping her children off at my house whenever she needed some time. It felt awkward, since I wasn't running a daycare, but I let it happen, unable to establish a healthy boundary around my time and energy. When people needed me, I'd always showed up. *Stay strong*, I'd tell myself. *Do more, faster, better.*

"I Need *Something*"

Abundant yogi. That was what the Facebook ad said.

Kris, the abundant yogi, was wearing ripped jeans in her photo. I couldn't get enough of her hopeful and inspiring message. Weeks after signing up for her email list, I got on a call with her. Almost immediately, I was hooked. Her coaching program cost over a thousand dollars, and even when it was broken down into three installments, the size of each payment was well outside my budget. Determined, I called Bryan to ask for his credit card number because my card was already maxed out.

"What are you buying?" he asked.

"It doesn't matter," I replied. "I'm desperate. I need *something*."

Kris's coaching was around creating an online product. At the time, I didn't have a community, so while I implemented every step as she prescribed, when all was said and done, I didn't sell a single product. However, during my coaching with her, I also had other homework—pleasure prescriptions, she called them. Bit by bit, she was introducing me to the idea of self-care, trying to get me to acknowledge that I, all by myself, mattered.

It felt exciting and oh-so necessary, but also awkward. I remember being in the backyard one day, reading *Mama Gena's School of Womanly Arts*. Just sitting and reading, that was my pleasure prescription for the week. As I tried to focus on the words in front of me, which were encouraging me to take care of myself in not one, but many important ways, it became suddenly clear to me that I didn't actually have to feel like crap all of the time. Yet almost as soon as I'd had that thought, I began worrying about how I'd be judged. What would people think if they saw me taking care of myself? Would they assume I was neglecting my children? Assuming that was true, I then felt an almost crushing wave of guilt overcome me. How could I even consider taking care of myself when my children needed me?

As much as I resisted taking care of myself, though, being given permission to do yoga, meditate, and try other things simply for the sake of feeling good gave me hope. I began to notice my thoughts, and to make a conscious effort to reorient my thinking in positive directions. For the first time in my life, I was finding out what it felt like to guide my thoughts away from the pressure to be the person other people wanted me to be and toward how I wanted to feel.

Shaking Things Up

While my coach was prescribing regular doses of pleasure, self-care, and self-compassion, my co-workers at the office were eating junk food, suffering physically, and giving their clients little to no compassion. Feeling like the health and wellness world had a lot to offer these women, I approached a supervisor about organizing a simple, informative wellness fair in the lunchroom at work. I would do it in my own time, I explained, and make sure it didn't interfere with my work. My assumption was that my supervisors, and eventually my co-workers, would be interested in feeling better, which would directly influence their work and ultimately benefit the company—that they would appreciate the opportunity to learn more.

Instead, my idea was met with stupefied disbelief. "Why would you want to do *that*, Heather?" was followed by "You're too soft, Heather" and "You'll never survive here, Heather." I made another attempt or two but eventually had to abandon the project altogether.

Running, Always Running...at 3 a.m.

The more disillusioned I became with social work and the culture of negativity that dominated the system, the more time and energy I poured into my side business. Eager to transform my career, I completed every action step prescribed by my coach. It shocked me that so many of the women going through the same coaching program were taking little to no action. *Don't you want to change your life?* I remember thinking. They seemed as dissatisfied with their careers as I was with mine. Their unwillingness to make progress made no sense to me. It was one of the first times I noticed that the panic that propelled me into perpetual activity—always going faster and doing more—could have the opposite effect and paralyze others.

The only thing I'd ever known how to do was survive, no matter what, always doing more and acknowledging as few of my emotions as possible. Now that I had two boys, taking action wasn't just an innate propensity, it was a non-negotiable necessity. I was unstoppable: a mom on a mission. Yet the way I was living, the pace I was trying to keep, wore on me. Desperate for more energy, patience, and time, I decided to adopt better habits and begin each day with a green smoothie. It was a positive change, but one that was quickly sabotaged by the fact that I often forgot to eat for hours afterward.

With my credit card maxed out, our finances increasingly stretched, and my career in social work feeling too stifling to sustain, I walked around in a controlled state of panic most of the time. My anxiety got so severe, I struggled to stay still. Eventually, it grew so intense, I'd get on the treadmill in our house at 3 a.m., too wired to sleep and too exhausted not to do something—anything—that would help me fall asleep. One stride at a time, I tried to burn off my anxiety, to tire my body out just enough to feel even a few hours of peace. It helped, but still, there was something bigger, less obvious, and far deeper begging for my attention.

The upside of my overscheduled life was that I could no longer deny how pressed for time I really was. When friends asked me if they could stop by, I agreed, provided they could help me make a green smoothie, hold Calvin, or whatever else I needed at any given moment. That was helpful, of course, but looking back, it was a lot like putting a Band-Aid on a broken arm.

Dissecting the Culture of Self-Sacrifice

Whenever I mentioned how exhausted I felt, I heard the same reply, "You've got young ones at home. *Of course* you're tired." Desperate for new ideas and solutions, I searched online, only to find mommy bloggers semi-joking about "mommy juice" and "wine o'clock."

At one point, I noticed a social media post from a famous billionaire entrepreneur, who's also a mom, bemoaning her perpetual exhaustion while essentially blaming it on mother-hood. I wasn't just disheartened, I was infuriated. She seemed like an empowered businesswoman, yet she, too, was buying into the idea that motherhood is about chaos and suffering. This idea is so deeply etched into our definition of what a "good" mother is, that no amount of money or status or out-side help can solve it. I remember seeing her post and thinking, *Is buying into this culture of self-sacrifice really the only way to be a "good" mother? Is mental, emotional, or physical depletion really all there is for us, as moms?*

Even while navigating my days consumed by guilt about not doing enough for my own kids—no matter what I did, it never felt like enough—I felt increasingly overwhelmed by how our broader culture was positioning motherhood as a kind of torture. The message was clear—if you weren't per-petually exhausted or in constant, desperate need of caffeine and/or wine, you must not be doing enough. If you weren't sacrificing your own needs and desires for your kids, you were failing. Being a "good" mother caused exhaustion, maybe even required it. It was fine to complain about it, even joke about it, provided you understood that this is what a "good" mother does.

The more aware I became of this message, the more I noticed it. Years earlier, a woman I looked up to told me that I needed to buy the cheaper shampoo now that I was a mother of two. I'd done as she suggested and bought the less expensive shampoo, only to find it disappointing and my hair lacklus-ter. My hair has always been my beauty fun zone, something I enjoy that makes me feel like me. I remember wondering, *Why should I sacrifice something that makes me feel so good just to save ten or twelve bucks?* I soon went back to buying the "expen-sive" shampoo and, for once, didn't feel guilty about "treating" myself.

However, that one tiny act of rebellion couldn't overpower the million others that did center on self-sacrifice. Drawing energy from what felt like sparse reserves, I kept on working, teaching, and giving more, desperate for validation from the world around me. As I dove deeper into the health and wellness world, I secretly yearned to be the "perfect" marathon-running mom, the meditation-and-green-juice mom, with her own business too. I was trying, but also failing. As my meditation classes grew in size, I still couldn't overcome my anxiety enough to make a green smoothie from scratch. Having grown up in a house where the kitchen was primarily for food storage, rather than actual cooking, the mere thought of shopping for ingredients and making a green smoothie for myself, in my own kitchen, felt impossibly overwhelming.

Taking a Step

Even as I became more passionate about taking a stand for mothers who were taking care of themselves in whatever ways they could, there was no denying that I still wasn't happy. Physically, mentally, and emotionally, I felt weighed down by a heavy blanket of misery that began morphing into a quiet, yet undeniable, sense of desperation. Was this what motherhood was about? If so, I didn't want it. I'd never wanted to feel this way. There were so many days when I badly wanted to break down in tears, too weary at a deep soul level to "make it all work" for another single second. My kids were amazing creatures, and both of them had fully captured my heart, yet secretly I wondered how much more I had to give. Even as I grew more passionate about our need to self-nurture, I wore my fatigue like a badge of honor, a sign that I was at least in the running to become a "good" mother.

This feeling of always being too many steps behind only grew as Calvin did. The closer he got to becoming a toddler, the more energy he had. The more he could move, the more he insisted he needed to. He was in nonstop, full-on action from the moment he opened his eyes to whenever he finally closed them.

Prior to this point in my life, I'd never been a morning person. I wasn't in the habit of jolting out of bed or going from zero to a hundred in seconds, yet with Calvin, that seemed mandatory. It rattled me deeply, fraying my nerves and clipping my patience. As someone who's always been highly sensitive to noise and energy, I felt perpetually out of sync with how fast and loud my home life was becoming.

Finally, I decided I'd had enough. Starting every day in a panic was wearing on me. Bryan often received the brunt of my anxiety; I was beginning to resent starting every day off on the wrong foot. Now fully immersed in the online health and wellness world, I'd heard several industry leaders talk about the importance of adhering to a morning routine. It was time for me to create one for myself.

That decision to make what amounts to a simple daily change has proven hugely valuable. Over time, it has also become a habit that I still rely on to start my day. As with nearly everything, from eating to exercise, meditation, and more, I do best when I let myself be flexible. I'm not rigid about habits, and I don't do well when I try to stick to one routine for too long. That may mean that I'm really into meditating for a period of weeks or months, only to discover one day that journaling is calling to me instead.

While the idea of staying open to your new yearnings and desires may seem appealing, in a culture that often defines success as always doing more, better, my need for flexibility can feel, or even look like, failure. Am I less of a meditator because I don't practice every single day? Am I less of a runner because sometimes I go on yoga kicks, and less of a yogi because I sometimes prefer to go running? Am I less disciplined because my morning routine on Thursday may differ from what it was on Monday?

As I've renegotiated my relationship with the idea and practice of my morning routine in the years since beginning one, I've had to accept the fact that my idea of a successful morning routine means having one at all. To me the goal is to create mornings that nurture me spiritually, emotionally, and physically. How that happens, and how that changes from one day to the next, no longer bothers me.

Whether you do better with this more flexible approach or a more consistent one, I encourage you to begin looking at your own mornings. How can you make the start of your day feel more fulfilling?

Tracking Your Progress

From this point forward, as you begin your journey of self-discovery, I highly recommend using a journal, as it will allow you to track your thoughts, emotions, and progress. Feel free to use a printed journal or an app like Day One.

Reinvent Your Mornings Challenge

Whether your mornings are a thorn in your side or could simply use more of your attention, my challenge for you is to make them feel nourishing and rejuvenating. If you feel too pressed for time to do anything new or different in the morning, begin by waking up five minutes earlier for the next week. If you need more time after that, wake up ten minutes earlier the following week, and so on, until your mornings feel relaxing and enjoyable.

For the first week, when you're waking up five minutes earlier, pick one activity—meditating, journaling, or something else—and do that each morning, during your extra five minutes.

Try using my 30-Day A.M. Routine Planning Chart, which guides you in how to gradually turn your morning routine into a grounding ritual that starts your day on a good note. One morning at a time, it supports you in taking small amounts of additional time for yourself. For example, you might add one extra minute to your meditation practice each day or each week. You also might begin on day one by writing one sentence about how you want to feel and gradually work up to writing a single paragraph about how you want to feel. These kinds of incremental changes are often more sustainable than trying to adopt an "ideal" morning routine right away.

Go to dyingtobeagoodmother.com to download my free 30-Day A.M. Routine Planning Chart.

4

Really Seeing Children

ALMOST AS SOON AS Sammy walked into the room, I sensed that he was trying to tell me something. It was our first meeting, and he was clearly searching for someone he could trust, someone who would listen to what he had to say without telling him what and who he "should" be.

Like many of the kids in the system, Sammy had been classified as having "behavioral issues," but from the moment I met him, I saw something different. He had this incredible light that brightened the room. He was also funny, entertaining, and disruptive. He wasn't big on following rules, so if I told him he could have two pieces of candy, he'd try to get three. That didn't bother me. In fact, I respected his scrappy attitude; it showed his resilience. But it also showed me that if I didn't listen, Sammy would make sure I "heard" him by using behavior to get my attention.

That light I saw in Sammy was often masked. His life had been far too hard for far too long. He'd been through things that no child can easily understand or process—abuse, neglect, abandonment—and he wasn't quick to trust the adults in his life as a result. I didn't blame him or hold it against him. Trust is vulnerable, a privilege that must be earned.

Being disruptive was how he got attention. It was also how he figured out which, if any, adults would truly and deeply listen to what he was trying to say to the world. Knowing that Sammy was testing me, I made a point of not approaching him the way that most adults he'd known had—armed with rules and expectations that he "had to" meet. Instead, I focused on creating connection.

I knew I had to communicate with him on his terms and let him know that I accepted him as he was. It took time, but little by little, as I gained his trust, I began to set some boundaries, always making sure to reward him for his respect. The more he trusted me, the more boundaries I could create. There were very real limits to how hard and fast I could push him, though. A single misstep on my part—one failure to make him feel seen and heard—and all of the work I'd done to earn his trust might suddenly be undone.

That was true with all the kids I worked with in my job. I had to prioritize my respect for them above and beyond the rules, above and beyond what I was "supposed" to do. How I interacted with each of them varied depending on their personality and willingness to engage on any given day. When kids were defensive, I'd immediately back off. That was my way of saying, *I see you and your need for space. I'm here, but I also respect the boundary you're laying down.* The kids who reacted to the trauma they'd survived by going inward sometimes wanted to paint or write. When they let me, I joined them. Other times, I'd simply sit with kids in silence, making sure not to project any judgment on them or their desire not to connect in any outward way.

The more time I spent with these kids, the more I appreciated and respected them. They'd been through so much and had had so few of their basic needs—stability, safety, nurturing, love, food, and reliable shelter—met. At one point a senior staffer at the office remarked that I had a "special something" around connecting with the children in the system. It wasn't a coincidence. I'd experienced feeling unseen and misunderstood throughout my own childhood. When at a very young age the world tells you that you don't matter, your shame grows so acute and so sharp that all you want to do is vanish. Very quickly you learn to keep your pain to yourself. You figure out that daring to speak your true feelings is often misinterpreted as a reason for people to try to "fix" you. It's exhausting, so you stop speaking and instead use behavior as a means of communicating your complicated emotions to a world that's not interested, a world that's quick to judge and slow to care enough to actually listen.

It's a searing pain to grow up with. Not wanting other children to have to suffer in those ways, I became the adult I needed as a child.

Like many of the children I was now overseeing in my job, I, too, had struggled in school. Rebellious by nature, I constantly asked why we were learning this or that, and why I had to hand in an assignment that seemed pointless to me. My curiosity had often been interpreted as disrespect and viewed as a sign that I'd never succeed in life. From a young age, I, like the children I was now observing, had heard that I wasn't smart enough or worthy enough to succeed in school or in life.

These children didn't just speak to me; on some deeper level they *were* me. I could relate to them because in ways that weren't obvious but still felt very personal, I'd been like them.

Trying to Slow the Downward Spiral

Once children were removed from their families and put into foster care, they were monitored and assessed. Their backgrounds varied. Sometimes there had been abuse, neglect, addiction issues, and more. Being put into foster care was something that happened for a lot of different reasons; the longer I worked at my job, the clearer it became that while every one of these kids had been through trauma, each case was also unique.

In spite of the many different circumstances these kids had been forced to withstand, they were universally evaluated according to their behavior. If they "acted out" in any way, they were labeled as having "behavioral issues." When their behavior was judged as "disruptive," they were typically punished, often by taking away something they liked or revoking some privilege.

If a child's behavior continued to become more challenging, the kids were often categorized as "defiant" and put through the system, many of them medicated along the way. If the undesirable behavior(s) continued, they were kicked out of the institution they were in and placed in high-security group homes. If those group homes were unable to handle them, their medications were typically increased, sometimes repeatedly. As the drugs in their system compounded, a lot of them started to appear mentally unsound. Some were then diagnosed with schizophrenia or bipolar disorder, destined for mental health facilities where they would essentially be prisoners for much of their lives.

I was continually amazed, and not in a good way, that psychology professionals were so quick to hand out diagnoses and medications that would ultimately amount to a life sentence to children who were so clearly in need of attention, caring, and compassion. The compounding of mind-altering drugs in their systems likely limited their mental and physical functioning over time. Plus, all of them had been traumatized and placed into unknown circumstances with unknown people.

Often, this happened very quickly, so they'd live in one place in the morning and a different place that same night. Expecting anyone to adjust to that kind of upheaval, often repeatedly, especially on top of pre-existing trauma, is a lot to ask. For children, who have no control over their circumstances and limited capacity to understand what's happening and why, it's even more overwhelming. Typically, though, none of this was taken into consideration. Instead, there was a laser-like focus on how the kids were behaving, and minimal, if any, consideration of how they were feeling.

I remember one time when a young child was having a massive tantrum. As my co-workers and I discussed what to do, I asked if I could try to settle him. They agreed, so I entered the room where he was screaming and throwing things. I sat down, making a point of not judging him or his behavior. "It's okay," I told him. "No one's going to hurt you. You're fine. I've got you." I repeated things like this as he continued to make noise and kick things. Eventually, he calmed down. "What happened?" I asked. He wouldn't tell me. I nodded and said "okay."

I'd brought crayons into the room with me, which eventually caught his attention. We began drawing, and he asserted himself, insisting on taking charge of the drawing. Knowing how little about his life he'd been able to control, I nodded. "You can control the drawing. That's fine." He kept drawing calmly.

I wish I could say that I changed that child's life, that he's now fine and was able to grow up in a stable and loving home. I don't know where he is now, or what his life's been like. What I did see in him, and in many others like him, was how desperately he needed what the system was failing to provide—love, nurturing, and stability. He needed to be seen, heard, and understood, rather than judged, medicated, and relocated over and over again.

Recording Trauma

Part of my job was sitting behind a glass wall and observing kids with their parents, often while they were actively under-going trauma. These were families at risk, and more often than not, the moments I had to observe were riddled with the kind of complexity that's hard to wrap your mind around.

One of my most haunting moments behind the glass was when a child was visiting with her father, who had been accused of sexually abusing her. Far too young to defend her-self or speak up, she sat there, near the parent who had violated her, as I watched, equally unable to help her. (The case was in court at the time, so there wasn't sufficient evidence to pre-vent the visitation.) I'll never forget sitting there, feeling utterly powerless to protect this little child. All I was allowed to do was watch and record their interactions. It felt wrong, completely against my most basic nature. I'd studied social work to help people, but what I was actually doing was helping to perpetu-ate a system I didn't believe in.

There were boys, too, who had been molested, and some-times fathers who made inappropriately sexual comments to me in front of their children. Every time I worked my shift, I witnessed the debilitating effects of multi-generational pov-erty, hopelessness, trauma, addiction, mental health issues, and more. However heartbreaking these children's circum-stances were, I was expected to stay professional, which is another way of saying emotionally detached. Not taking our clients' pain home was expected, even applauded, but it was also the one thing I couldn't do.

Looking around, I was shocked to realize that I was the exception among my peers at the office, who seemed to digest their role as monitor with far less resistance and anguish. Many of my co-workers resorted to indifference, as well as judgment, often saying harsh things about their clients instead of empathizing with them. It was how they survived, I knew, but it was also against my basic nature.

After being exposed to many of these situations, I finally cracked one day and did exactly what I wasn't supposed to do—choose my client over the system and its many rules. On that particular day, I was asked to oversee a mom and her son. This woman and her husband seemed to live a "nice" life in a middle-class neighborhood, but they were being investigated for domestic violence. She was clearly mortified to be in the system as a family at risk. I did what I had to do and laid down the rules, which gave her a specified amount of time to stay with her son before he was returned to his foster home. She delayed repeatedly, desperate to stay with her child. Finally, I had no choice but to call for supervision. While someone else held her back, I had to tear the boy from his mother's arms while he screamed and screamed. It was the first time I'd had to act against my own instincts as a mother, look this woman in the eyes and say "He must go" as I removed him from her care.

He was being taken away from her. Her heart was being ripped from her arms, and not surprisingly, her basic human instinct to protect her cub soon kicked in. Of course she was going to attack, and she did that with her words. My heart broke; I was a mother too. Sure, there were decisions and mistakes she had made that led to this moment, but still, this didn't feel like a time for judgment.

My heart racing, tears welling in my eyes, I closed the door behind me and stood facing her as she projected her fear, anger, and frustration onto me. While she unloaded, all I could think about is how would I feel if I were in her shoes. And I knew I would have acted and reacted in the exact same ways.

When she was quiet, I empathized with her pain, acknowledged her courage, and let her know that I was listening, that I wasn't judging her, and that she could and should keep fighting. I hugged her, knowing there was no more I could do, profoundly aware that I couldn't give her what she wanted and needed—her son—and then led her out.

We don't always agree with the choices people make, and sometimes their decisions do lead to children being taken out of the home. Is the system flawed? Yes, but what system isn't? Regardless of the details of that mother's particular situation, she taught me something that day. She showed me that despite the legal action that was being taken to protect her children, I could stand with her as a woman, a mother, and a sister seeking connection with compassion and without judgment. That was all I could give her in that moment. It couldn't take away her pain or give her back the son we'd just ripped from her arms, but I could at least give her the respect, kindness, and consideration we all deserve.

Yearning to Disrupt the Status Quo

Every time I delivered a status report to my supervisor, I made a point of highlighting how I could help my clients. To me that seemed like the most basic and essential part of my job. Most of my clients were victims of systemic and cultural prejudice, if not racially then socioeconomically. Almost without exception, they were being shown few, if any, ways to defend and help themselves. It felt inhuman not to try to help them live better lives. However, each time I mentioned how I intended to help a client, my supervisor would respond with something like, "Oh, Heather, you'll never survive here." Long before I realized it myself, she saw my inability to establish the boundaries I would need to continue doing the social work that was breaking my heart a little more each day.

Instead of spending time getting to know and understand my clients, I was supposed to do things like lecture them on how to parent. One day, I was charged with talking to an Indigenous family with multiple children. They were well known on the streets, and widely considered to be dangerous. As I sat there, instructing them in how to parent, I felt both afraid and ashamed. I didn't know them, their children, or their culture. Nor had I experienced the countless traumas they'd survived. How could I possibly understand their experience? And how was it my place to tell them how to raise their own children?

The harder I tried, the more out of sync I felt with my job. Without question, I felt my most out of alignment and disconnected from my purpose when I did what I was supposed to. Only when I broke the rules and followed my gut did I feel any relief and reassurance that by being myself, I could make a positive difference in people's lives.

Mama, I See You

The moment the words were out of my mouth, I could feel her emotional wall go up. "You're going to leave me like all the others," she said, her voice quivering with anger and maybe fear too.

I was a student and my time with this particular client was up. I had to go. During our months together, I'd convinced her that she could go back to school and make something of herself. I'd believed in her, and perhaps for the first time, she'd begun to believe me and invest in the hope and possibility of a different future. But now I was leaving, and my departure wasn't as simple as saying goodbye. For her it was killing off her hope and her potential to turn herself and her life into something she and her children could feel proud of.

As I got to know a few of the children in the system, I also started to get acquainted with some of their mothers. This particular client had young twins and had already had her eldest child taken away from her and placed in foster care. She herself was a crown ward, someone who grew up in the system and was released at age eighteen without ever having been adopted. From our first meeting, something about her made me want to do whatever I could to help her. Over a period of months, I warmed my way into her heart, often telling inappropriate jokes that helped her let her guard down.

Having partially relied on government aid to get myself through school, I knew that as a crown ward she would qualify for considerably more substantial aid than I'd gotten. Sensing that she wanted to change her life, I began encouraging her to go back to school. That would empower her to protect her twins, and perhaps even prove to her eldest child that she'd fought to get her back by making something of herself.

When I reported all of this back to my supervisor, she scolded me for putting "false hope" in this woman, who, she asserted, was "stupid." I was infuriated and disheartened, but still too young and naive to see that the social work career I was aspiring to would never be a fit for me; that my supervisor was in fact right about the false hope part. It wasn't because this woman was "stupid," though. It was because no one had ever believed in her or taught her how to believe and invest in herself.

Assuming I was doing what was best, instead of heeding my supervisor's counsel, I'd persevered and walked my client through the school registration process. She got hopeful for a while, and I felt excited about making a difference in her life. She successfully completed the registration process, but then the day came when I had to tell her I was leaving, that I was being reassigned. Without me there to guide her, I suddenly saw that the chances of her following through and going to school long enough to earn a degree were slim. The fact was, too many people had abandoned her, and she hadn't ever received enough support and caring to know how to care for herself and, in turn, her children. That was all clear to me now, but tragically, my clarity wasn't doing her any favors.

It's easy to judge mothers like her, especially in the "picture perfect" parenting culture we now see on social media. The truth is, though, she, and most of the mothers I worked with later as part of my job, loved their children deeply. They were all doing their best in the midst of incredibly painful and difficult circumstances. Even with so much hardship in their lives and so few reasons to hope for a positive outcome, one mother after another would show up to her meeting with a social worker, knowing that her failure to appear could result in losing custody of her children. Even the mothers who said unkind things to their children weren't being intentionally mean; most of them had lived through more trauma than any human can handle and were simply trying to protect their children from the same fate. The only way they knew how to do that was by scaring and shaming their children into obedience.

The Red, Yellow, and Green Zones

Imagine yourself driving a car. As you approach a red light, you stop and wait for the light to turn green. When it finally does, you go and keep going until you see a yellow light, so you slow down and prepare to stop.

We recognize and respect these signals when we're driving yet override similar cues from the body. Why don't we listen to what the body is trying to tell us?

At some point, after working with these families, I started talking about "the zones." I honestly don't remember when the whole concept even came to me, but I began to notice, think, and talk about them with the clients I was now teaching and coaching outside of my job.

There was a clear pattern of emotional states that people operate from. I began referring to them as the three zones—red, yellow, and green.

The Red Zone

When we're in the red zone, we're so revved up emotionally—so overcome by big emotions like anger, fear, and shame—that we're unable to process information or communicate effectively. When we're in the red zone, we usually know it. In fact, in addition to feeling it emotionally, we may also experience our heightened emotions physically through sweaty palms, rapid heartbeat, and more.

In the red zone, we're most likely to lash out and say and do things we later regret. These aren't actions we've thought through—they're knee-jerk responses to the intense emotions we're feeling in the moment. In this place it's best for us to avoid engaging in discussions with others because we're too riled up to express ourselves or take in what other people are saying. Instead, this is a time to step back and do whatever we need to do to digest and process our emotions.

The Yellow Zone

The next level down from the red zone is the yellow zone. This one can be harder to identify, both in ourselves and others. It's where we're bothered, even agitated, but not necessarily acting on it. Children and adults alike may be in their yellow zone after a long day of school or work, or after something unsettling has happened. One of the challenges of the yellow zone is that we may not even notice when we ourselves are in it—until we suddenly tip over into the red zone and do something that we later regret. Seeing when we, and others, are in the yellow zone takes effort, practice, and focus.

People often tell me that they or their children don't have yellow zones, that they go from green to red, "just like that." I've literally never found this to be the case. It can seem like we, or others, skip the yellow zone only because it was too subtle to notice, or we were too distracted to pick up on yellow zone cues. Nonetheless, we do pass through the yellow zone on our way to red.

Yellow Zone Cues

Before the red zone kicks in...

- **Mind:** Tired, fatigued thoughts, anxious thoughts, overwhelmed

- **Body:** Sweaty palms, racing heart, stomachache, tightness or tension, fatigue

- **Emotions:** Impatient, agitated, anger beginning to rise, feeling triggered, feeling depleted, wanting to escape or pretend everything's fine when it's not

Another tricky part about the yellow zone is that we can stay in it for hours, days, even weeks. Let's say something upsetting happens—maybe we get bad news, or someone says something that feels passive-aggressive. Either because we're too busy to focus on it, or we'd simply rather not think about it, we end up simmering silently in the yellow zone for days or weeks. Then one day, we see that person. Everything is fine at first, but then they say something irritating, and immediately we're set off. To the other person, we may seem to have gone from green to red "just like that," but in reality, we've been in the yellow zone for days, without even fully realizing it ourselves.

The Green Zone

The green zone is a much easier place to be. It's where we're calm, open, and in a good place to engage with others and generally enjoy life. This is the ideal place to start a new practice, whether it's a new morning routine or meditation, a new kind of exercise... (All of these habits are useful in every zone, but they're often easier to start when we're in the green zone.)

Over the years, as I've presented these zones to various clients and groups, some have compared the concept to emotional states of regulation. To be honest, I've never studied that; the concept of these zones just came to me as I was working with people in my job and in my classes. Regardless, using the zones to guide decision-making has been profound for me, my family, and my clients.

One day, after presenting the concept of the three zones at a school, the principal came up to me. "That was a total game changer," he said enthusiastically. "Don't try to solve problems in your red zone." He was right. By learning to disengage when we're in our red zone, we can avoid a lot of unnecessary conflict, drama, and misunderstanding. By mastering all three zones, we can transform how we relate to ourselves, our lives, and others.

Reconciling with Resistance

After the wellness fair idea withered with my colleagues, I realized that my true desire was to teach meditation to the kids I worked with. As soon as I presented that idea to supervisors, it was shut down immediately and completely. This time, I'd gotten a firm no. That much was clear.

Feeling dejected and deflated, I continued to struggle with the realities of my job. I was surrounded by so much need—in my clients, their children, and my co-workers—but also by equal, if not greater, resistance around investing in any kind of positive change. I felt stuck and overwhelmed by my desire to help people. The deeper I connected with these families, the clearer it became that the system was peddling hopelessness. The people in the system had simply suffered from too much trauma to fight back, and no one was willing to support them in creating the change that they badly needed.

On a personal level, these realizations hit harder than I expected. Yes, my doubts about my future in social work had been mounting for some time, but still, each new judgment and rejection stung. My co-workers and supervisors really had been right; I *wasn't* built for social work. My desire to make a positive impact on people's lives was too deeply rooted. The fact was, I didn't want to become indifferent or callous to the suffering of others. But how could I leave my clients behind? My guilt felt intense and unrelenting.

Ultimately, admitting that I wasn't meant for social work felt unavoidable, as well as empowering and terrifying. What if I couldn't make it on my own either? Truth be told, my side business was growing, but also costing more than it was making. I wasn't just not earning money. I was accumulating more debt that we could possibly manage, and there was no indication that I could succeed enough to reverse that trend.

PART II

From Darkness Comes Light

5

From Chaos to Control

'D OCCASIONALLY SEE clients getting on or off a bus at this one stop near my house. The longer I stayed in social work, the more that fact terrified me. I worried about safety, especially when I was with my children, and then I felt guilty about feeling afraid.

It was no secret that I'd grown fond of some of the children and mothers I worked with in the system, but that same system was also doing my clients no favors. Whether I liked it or not, I was part of that broken and biased machine. At some point my clients might begin to blame me for that, and really, why wouldn't they? No one had ever looked out for them. My attempts to advocate for their needs had been rebuffed repeatedly by my supervisors, which meant that in my clients' eyes I would eventually become one more person who'd failed them. It felt shameful avoiding the bus stop, but it also felt like the right decision. I had to protect my children.

However, the truth was that my children weren't suffering because we lived near that bus stop. Nor were they feeling threatened by my clients or co-workers. As Logan proceeded into his second year of school (senior kindergarten, or SK, in

Canada), our home life unraveled a little more, a little faster, with each passing week. In actual fact it was I, their mother, who was the biggest threat to their well-being and happiness.

"Unacceptable"

By the end of Logan's JK year, I'd begun to hear from his teachers. He was acting out, they reported, unable to adhere to "simple" routines like sitting for thirty minutes during circle time. It was a far cry from the reports I'd gotten just a year earlier. At the preschool Logan had attended before JK, the teachers seemed to take the children's actions and reactions in stride. Whereas there his energy and fidgeting had been seen as normal, now those same characteristics were being described in severe, judgmental terms. Logan's behavior, his teachers reported, was "unacceptable."

I'm sure I had to attend parent-teacher meetings, although I don't specifically remember them. What I do remember is noticing the behaviors his teachers were describing also playing out at home. It made me anxious and frustrated. I couldn't understand why his teachers couldn't relate to his behavior. Wasn't it normal for a four- or five-year-old? But if he was the only child having these issues, as his teachers seemed to be implying, then why couldn't he follow his teachers' instructions? Was I missing something?

As the school year progressed, the teachers' comments grew more serious. They insisted that "something was wrong," emphasizing that "testing was needed." There were multiple mentions of ADD and ADHD, and an increasingly clear message that Logan's so-called behavior was my problem. I needed to fix it, fix him, and by extension my parenting, and fast.

Feeling completely unsupported, I did what so many mothers do—I went into overdrive. Accepting the premise that his "behavior" was problematic, I resolved to fix it, and in the process, fix him.

In between my work shift, my side hustle teaching meditation, and caring for Logan and his rambunctious baby brother, I began to devise learning activities and games for Logan. After school each day, we'd come home, have a snack, and spring into action. With Calvin on my hip, his little body squirming and kicking tirelessly, I'd give Logan some kind of academic activity. "Let's sing the alphabet song!" I'd announce in an upbeat tone of voice. Being in Ontario, Canada, he needed to be able to recite and identify all of the letters in English and French, so A (English) was also *ah* (French) and B, *beh*. The same applied to numbers, writing, counting, and so on. There was a lot of work to do, and once I'd harnessed my get-it-done energy, there was virtually no stopping me.

At one point I hired a high school student to tutor Logan. At my request, after school one day we all met at a nearby playground, where I proceeded to paste the letters of alphabet, in French, all around the jungle gym. At my prompting the tutor was to have Logan find *ah*, then *beh*, and so on, all over the climbing structure.

Wasn't this what any aspiring "good" mother would do—devise learning activities that worked with her child's fidgety, hyperactive nature?

Logan was too young to understand that the activity was academic in nature, but still he made sure to have his say. He found a letter, maybe two, before promptly schooling me in Playground 101: when at the playground, children play. Off he went, not remotely interested in finding C (*ceh*) or any letters after it.

Different versions of this scenario played out day after day, week after week. Each time some new plan to "fix" Logan's behavior and learning backfired, I felt my frustration amplifying, morphing faster each time into a hot, untenable anger.

The True Meaning of "Acting Out"

Even then, before Logan was old enough to understand that I was trying to "fix" his behavior, he was communicating with me in the same way that the children at my work were trying to communicate with the adults in their lives—through how he was acting. Given how focused I was on children's behavior as a form of communication in my work, you'd think I would have noticed Logan's many attempts to convey his needs—but I didn't, at least not at first.

At work I intuitively understood that defiance from a child was often a way for children to communicate unmet needs and re-establish boundaries that were too often being ignored or disregarded. With my meditation students and their parents, I got that being fidgety and restless was how children met their own energetic needs. Ironically, when I was at home with Logan, all of this knowing, all of this ability to connect with children on their level and in their "language," was quickly overshadowed by the increasingly overwhelming, often contradictory, echo of my inner critic. *You're failing as a mother, Heather. All you do is yell. . . . Why won't he do what I'm asking? What's wrong with my child?*

I felt stressed and worried in almost equal measure. Could he have other cognitive or developmental issues? The possibilities were numerous, and as weeks passed, my mind spit out one worst-case scenario after another. Was Logan's inability to follow rules at school my fault? Did he have some undiagnosed condition? Was his "unacceptable" behavior a reflection of my bad parenting?

As the feedback from Logan's teachers grew more serious— "he needs testing" became an ongoing refrain for months that felt like years—I found myself tamping down a deep sense of shame. I'd been a low-income, unemployed teenager when I'd had Logan. Sure, I'd gotten scrappy and managed to get myself a university degree, but the fact was, he'd been born into less than ideal circumstances and to a father with chronic addiction issues, whom he'd never even met. Was this all my fault?

Hearing the teachers go on about his "issues," I worried about Logan, but also at least as much about myself. If something was "wrong," it had to be my fault somehow. Had I doomed my own child by getting pregnant as a teenager? Our life was more stable than it had been, but still, my side hustle was barely making money, and the pay from my job was measly. Bryan had a good job, but we were now shouldering so much debt, we basically still qualified as low income. Had my many unconventional decisions put my firstborn at a statistical disadvantage?

The shame and fear that was buried deep inside me seemed like more than I could handle, so I didn't try. Instead, I let myself remain emotionally deaf to Logan's behavioral communication. Even as I wholeheartedly accepted other children's need to move around and shift their focus during my meditation classes, I found Logan's inability to focus on academics after school increasingly unbearable. Why couldn't he just do what I was asking? How were the other children in his SK class able to sit still when he never could? And why was he falling behind academically?

More often than I wanted to admit, I lost my patience, resorting to angry yelling that backfired with Logan and left me feeling overwhelmed by a fresh dose of scalding shame. I had studied social work, as well as child development. Even my cynical supervisor had noted my ability to connect with children, yet here I was, unable to offer my own child the compassion and understanding I regularly gave to children I barely even knew.

Intellectually, I knew that my angry reactions could damage Logan's self-esteem. Yet emotionally, in the heat of the moment when Logan refused to follow my guidance, I was getting triggered on a level I struggled to control. He'd do something, or something would happen, and in an instant, I'd lose my mind and get very aggressive. In other words, I was spending a lot of time in my yellow zone, which also meant that I was moving into my red zone very quickly. With almost no warning, I'd begin shouting, and I was gritting my teeth so hard I started to worry that I'd lose them years before turning thirty.

One day, as this pattern reached another fever pitch, Logan hurled a toy across the living room. I was shocked, furious, and devastated. Anger, fear, and dread coursed through me. *Not this, not this, not this. This can't be what parenthood feels like,* I remember thinking. In that moment, even as my anger erupted, I knew something had to change.

Seeking Guidance, Finding Rebellion

Feeling fed up and exhausted, I went to Logan's pediatrician, hoping to get some of the guidance I wasn't getting from Logan's teachers. I also talked to the therapist I was seeing at the time. Neither of these professionals was alarmed, and both seemed sure that Logan's behavior was a phase, and a normal one at that.

While I still felt frustrated and unsupported, their input did feel validating. Since first hearing from Logan's teachers, I'd also grown my meditation classes, which now included occasional classes for mothers. When I closed the door and the other mothers began talking, the stories coming out of their mouths sounded eerily familiar. They, too, had heard from teachers about their children's behavior in class. They, too, were struggling to get their children to do simple things like sit still and listen. I wasn't alone after all. Logan was a normal, healthy five-year-old.

Very quickly, my perspective started to shift. The ongoing and increasingly severe drumbeat of criticism coming from the teachers had also simultaneously awakened my protective "mama bear" instincts, as well as my rebellious instincts. What was wrong with these teachers? Didn't they understand children at all? They had no right to treat Logan like a "problem" child!

It was teachers like Logan's, as well as other professionals who promoted fearmongering among parents, who were the real problem, I realized. Even as I had just barely come out of my own fog of judgment-induced shame and fear, I found myself feeling baffled by how quickly intelligent and well-informed parents like the mothers in my meditation classes were giving their power away to professionals who possessed so little true awareness.

Most of the time, the children were simply reacting through their behavior to how the adults were showing up. When adults came at them with judgment, fear, and shame, the children's behavioral responses might be anything from defiance and anger to indifference and ignoring. When adults showed up with patient, accepting energy, children were typically more open to guidance, including learning new ways to handle challenging situations.

Logan wasn't the "problem" child he was being made out to be. He was just communicating through his behavior, as young children do.

Avoiding the Diagnosis Trap

After months of hearing that "testing was needed," I still hadn't had Logan tested. Testing, his teachers had explained, would allow them to create an appropriate strategy for Logan. Their point was valid, but to a limited degree.

I now often coach mothers who tell me, "Oh, we're just waiting for the diagnosis." I usually reply, "That's fine. That's great, but no diagnosis will solve the problems that you're trying to address." With or without a diagnosis, parenting by yelling does not support a loving, trusting relationship. With or without a diagnosis, when parents regularly have the kinds of outbursts that once dominated my own parenting, there's some important relationship repair work to be done. No diagnosis can do that for you or your child.

To be clear, I do believe that strategy is important. We all need strategy in our lives. It helps us channel our energy productively—in our work, our relationships, and definitely in our parenting. Sometimes that strategy includes a diagnosis; at times it may even depend on one. However, as I exited the fog of shame, fear, and guilt about Logan and my own parenting, I began to realize that even the best strategy can only do 10 percent of the work.

The remaining 90 percent of the work happens when we, as parents, take time to engage in meaningful self-care. When we regularly carve out time to move the body and calm the mind, we can ask ourselves, how am *I* feeling? Instead of focusing solely on what others are doing, saying, and thinking, we can ask ourselves, how does this situation or solution feel *to me*? Even just on an intuitive level, we often know so much more than we give ourselves credit for. When we take even a little bit of time to get quiet and connect with our inner wisdom, we discover an entire world of ideas, feelings, and possibilities inside us. It's ultimately from that place that we can connect with our potential to thrive and grow through even the most challenging circumstances.

With this new perspective taking shape inside me, I made some decisions. Instead of pursuing testing, I listened to my inner guide and began meditating with Logan. He'd squirm and fidget within seconds of our first breaths, but instead of trying to "fix" his behavior, I let Logan be Logan. We practiced mindfulness in whatever small, brief ways we could, often trying new techniques and ways of being in the moment. It was basic, but he seemed to enjoy it.

Our joint meditation practice was a relief for me too. Finally, I was allowing myself to shed his teachers' judgments and focus on healing our relationship. It wasn't always easy, though. My urge to control the process and outcome was still inside me. It's just that by now, I had greater self-awareness. I was slowly but surely getting better at noticing my own thoughts and emotions. Day by day, I was practicing letting those urges come and go without them overtaking my actions and dictating my reactions. Because I was feeling more at ease, not being in complete control of our meditation practice felt less threatening. What mattered was that we were both learning (and relearning) how to be with our bigger emotions.

One Child, Many Parts

Have you ever wondered why a child flourishes in one school, but not in another? Have you ever seen your child behave cooperatively with one group and combatively or defiantly with another? Discovering a new solution can be as simple as looking at a situation from a different perspective. Instead of zeroing in on our children's behavior, we can look at the bigger picture and consider how different elements are interacting.

The Freedom to Just Be

Feeling increasingly out of alignment with my job, I often gave my shifts to co-workers who were eager for additional income. That meant that even the meager receipts from my side business were beginning to add up to more than the income from my job.

By this point, I'd moved my meditation classes out of our living room and into an event space at a nearby retail store. I offered to pay the store a rental fee, but they insisted I didn't need to. To this day I still wonder if they secretly felt sorry for me, but ultimately, I decided to accept the help and leave it at that.

Each children's meditation class typically ran for four weeks and cost around ten dollars per session per child. I'd tell friends and post flyers and get five or ten registrants each time I ran it. During each class, we'd begin in a circle. When I'd ask the children why they were there or what they wanted to learn, they'd often say things like, "Oh, I'm here because my parents say I'm too hyper," or, "I'm here because my mom says I have anxious thoughts." It was eye-opening realizing how many of these young children had already accepted the idea that they were flawed. At five and six years old, they'd taken on the belief that their emotions and behavior somehow needed fixing.

The more I saw this, the more I yearned to create a space where the children could be themselves. We practiced meditation some days, and on others we'd draw while listening to meditative music or pull oracle cards and talk. After class, one parent after another would come up to me and ask the same question—*Did you fix my child?* Given my experiences with Logan's teachers, I understood where these parents were coming from. They loved their children and ultimately wanted the best for them. However, they were also parenting from a place of fear and shame, trying to make their children fit into society's boxes and columns instead of allowing them to evolve in their own ways and on their own timeline.

Each time a parent asked this question, I would gently ask what was going on at home, and in an instant, I'd witness one parent after another visibly shut down. They needed to believe there was a perfect solution outside of themselves, and someone who knew how to implement it.

The teaching work lit me up like nothing else ever had, but in those moments I felt disheartened. So many well-meaning parents were too overwhelmed by their own emotions to open up to the idea that they, too, might be contributing to a dysfunctional dynamic at home.

My Experience, Mirrored

It was interesting undergoing this massive shift in my own perspective and beliefs while teaching my own child, and other children, how to meditate. The truth is, in spite of all the media about how meditation "increases focus" and "makes you more productive" and so on, the one thing you should always avoid with meditation is setting a goal. Sitting down to meditate to "fix your child," or for that matter, improve your focus or curb your cravings, et cetera, is the worst possible way to get started. Meditation is about being in the moment, with all the emotions and physical sensations, including discomfort, that we experience every day. While consistent meditation often leads to profound transformation, the practice itself should be about giving ourselves the space to just be, without any goal or outcome in mind.

No matter how much their parents cringed at hearing it, the children didn't need fixing. Most were just being children, developing exactly as they were meant to. In many cases they were reacting to the grown-ups around them.

Logan seemed to enjoy our meditation practice, and we both deepened our self-awareness and our capacity to feel, understand, and communicate. Like most kids, his ability to focus and sit still increased with age. He did slowly become more aware of how he was feeling, but that unfolded gradually, too, as it's meant to.

As we continued meditating together, it became so clear that Logan's biggest triggers were the people around him, including me. When I was disconnected from myself and highly reactive to my own emotions, he was more likely to have tantrums or get moody. In those moments, he was, as they say, "acting out," as in, acting out what he was feeling. When I felt out of control, he did, too, and his behavior put those confusing, overwhelming emotions on display.

As I gained mastery over my own mental state, I began parenting from this place of increased self-awareness. It was incredibly empowering. I didn't need to change anything about my child. Just by meditating and practicing observing my own emotions, I process them and show up differently. As it turned out, my learning to be present in any given moment was all Logan had ever needed.

All In, but Still on My Own

The more I meditated and taught meditation classes, the deeper I immersed myself in the personal development world. Louise Hay quickly became my new idol. I also hung on the wisdom of luminaries like Wayne Dyer, always engrossed in what I was learning, always thirsty for more; upon watching the movie *The Shift*, I felt so inspired, it seemed like I'd been spiritually and emotionally transported. *I'm IN!* I remember thinking. *Here, in this spiritual realm of infinite possibility, is where I belong.* It felt magical, rooting myself in this new way of being in the world.

Seeking out a new community that "got" this new me, I began hanging around the yoga crowd, both locally at the occasional studio class and also online. I also sometimes attended Reiki classes that were usually filled with seniors. I was amused being the only "young one" in the group but also didn't really care. I was there to learn more about energy healing. This world was my new world, my new love, and with or without people "like" me, I couldn't get enough. Even surrounded by people thirty and forty years older, I felt refreshed and renewed. Possibility was bubbling inside me. I could finally create a life that inspired, fulfilled, and energized me. In short, I was hooked.

At the same time, though, I began to notice that none of my new yoga friends were making any real money. They frequently gave away their time, energy, and expertise, or traded them for favors. Realizing this, I began to feel disheartened. Were these really my people? Weren't we, as spiritually evolving souls, supposed to be masters of manifesting? The whole idea was that our spiritual deposits could yield results that included real-world benefits, including money. Why were they failing at that part so miserably?

Finding My "In"

I wasn't yet willing or able to call my side hustle a business, but I did get that I needed to make money. We were in debt that was only growing. My money anxiety was always present, but I also didn't regret having spent the money that I had. Each new coach I'd worked with had made a huge difference in my mental health and my understanding of what it took to create and sell online products. Still, though, the balance on our credit card was higher than I'd ever imagined it would be. Making a lot more money was non-negotiable.

With all of the coaching and studying I was doing, I was noticing that people don't always buy what they need; it occurred to me that, sometimes, you have to appeal to your audience indirectly. Yearning to work with more mothers, I decided to offer a weekend-long day retreat. I called it Teach Your Kid to Meditate Teacher Training. I charged three hundred dollars per person, which was exponentially higher than any event fee I'd charged before. The pitch was that the parents would become experts, able to teach not only their own children, but also to host children's meditation classes themselves.

In theory I was offering to train people to become my competition, but my faith in the abundance of the Universe was also growing stronger, so I wasn't worried. I felt fairly sure that the mothers I would be training were seeking emotional and spiritual support more than aspiring to teach. Regardless, at the end of the event, I would present them each with a teacher certificate, which I printed at home.

When we sat down together on that first morning of the retreat, the floodgates opened almost immediately. One mother after another broke down about how much she felt like a failure. As I'd suspected it might, the weekend soon turned into a coaching and teaching weekend. These women's most pressing need wasn't learning how to teach; it was practicing meditation themselves so they could learn to be with the emotions they'd been running from, often for years.

Even though I focused more on coaching and practicing meditation than on teaching children how to meditate, the weekend was a great success. Realizing I could reach more mothers and make more money, I ran that same "teacher training" retreat several more times.

Mat Leave

With Calvin now a toddler and Logan a couple of years into school, I started feeling ready to have a third child. It would soon become the easiest pregnancy I'd ever had. It also brought an exciting, although scary, opportunity. According to Canadian law, I would have an entire year of maternity leave, aka, "mat leave." I wouldn't be paid during that year, but I was guaranteed to get my job back, if I wanted it, once the year was over.

That meant I had twelve months to turn my side hustle into a viable income. If I failed, I'd have to return to social work, knowing that the only way to survive there would be to participate in the collective hopelessness of "the system." I already knew I didn't have that in me.

Months before becoming pregnant with my third child, Felix, one of my supervisors had said something that surprised me. Recognizing my deep desire to make a difference in my clients' lives, she said, "Don't ever lose that part of yourself." I'd promised myself I wouldn't, which meant one thing—I had to find ways to make more money—a *lot* more money—from my side hustle. Pregnant or not, the pressure was on.

6

Wouldn't It Be Funny?

WITH FELIX NESTLED against me or chilling in a baby rocker that I'd nudge gently with my foot, I'd write marketing emails or give podcast interviews. Unless he was hungry, he was perfectly content to experience the world around him while I grew my coaching and teaching business. Truthfully, I'd have had a thousand Felixes, but that's not what life had in store for me. On a deep level I wasn't yet ready to acknowledge, I already kind of knew that.

My Little Angel

Each of my boys taught me something different. Logan taught me to live with purpose. Calvin taught me to laugh. Felix, who was born a few months before Calvin's third birthday, taught me to trust myself.

During my pregnancy with Felix, I'd meditated and used other personal development practices to become more mentally present and focused. It helped enormously; I felt calmer and more grounded than I ever had. My greatly improved mental health contributed very real results that included an easy pregnancy followed by an even easier birth.

Pooped Out

I was once again on all fours, but this time I was in my bed at home, a midwife on each side, when I had a sudden, strong urge. Unfortunately, that urge wasn't to give birth.

"I think I have to poop!" I said, a slight panic registering in my voice.

"No, that's the baby's head. You're going to give birth," a midwife calmly reassured me.

Instinctively, my insides contracted. This didn't feel like a baby. This felt like I needed to take a crap.

Just let it go, Heather. You've pooped thousands of times already. Just feel what you're feeling.

There's something especially vulnerable about letting yourself give in to the urge to poop when your ass is up in the air and you have an audience standing well within the drop zone. It was a level of visibility I hadn't prepared for. Thankfully, this time excluded Bryan, whom I'd asked to stay downstairs with my mom.

They've seen it all, Heather. Just let it go. All you have to do is poop.

Praying I'd never have to see these women again, I did what they asked. I pooped, and out came Felix. He was a quiet baby, so much so that I occasionally wondered if he was on the autism spectrum. Regardless, Bryan and I didn't push him to be verbal. He seemed happy just existing in our presence, even when our attention was divided, which happened often. Communicating with him non-verbally came easily, which made his reluctance to speak even more palpable. As a third child, he also did what youngest children do, learning early on how to mimic his brothers to get what he needed with minimal, if any, fuss.

His adaptability was a gift, even more so because of its timing. Since his first year of life was my "now or never" career year, having a baby who so easily fit into our lives and my schedule felt like the ultimate blessing. It also seemed like additional validation around the work I was doing. I was seeing results—for my clients and for myself and my family.

I loved being with Felix, having him so near me, but the fact was, I had very little downtime. While Logan was at school, Calvin and Felix increasingly had to fit in between the growing demands of my side hustle. Something or someone would have to give, but what or who would that be?

A Healthy Addiction

They say that when you're doing work that you truly love, you can forget to tend to basic needs like hunger and thirst. In many ways that summarizes my mat leave year with Felix. Every day I was filling my mind and soul with the richest, most nourishing food they'd ever had: the coaching and teaching work I was doing. It lit me up spiritually and intellectually like few things ever had.

Up until that point in my life, I'd harbored a belief that I had no real gifts; that nothing I could contribute was truly valuable. That feeling had gnawed at me for as long as I could remember, lulling me in my earlier years into the numbness of sleeping when what I'd actually needed was love, nurturing, and stimulation. That feeling had perhaps also drawn me to John, an addict who needed endless support and guidance, and may have once seemed like a human version of my "purpose."

When Logan was born, for the first time I'd begun to live with purpose, but my purpose had been Logan. Becoming a "good" mother would give me and my life worth and value, I'd told myself at the time. That idea had gotten me through school and into my first social work job, but as Logan had grown older and less dependent, new ideas and questions had begun to creep into my consciousness: *Being a mother isn't your only purpose, Heather. Who are you when you're standing by yourself, on your own two feet?*

Finally, during my mat leave year with Felix, as I dove deeper into the coaching and teaching work that felt like my life's purpose, the part of me that had believed I was worth so little began to heal. It was what I'd always desired and what I was almost endlessly willing to work for. So I did. Week after week, I buckled down and did everything in my power to get the word out, expand my network, grow my social media following and email list, and increase my visibility as a coach and teacher in whatever other ways I could.

Slowly but surely, my efforts began to bear fruit. I was asked to do interviews on various podcasts and attracted more followers on different platforms. It was exciting watching my client list expand and my revenue slowly rise along with it.

I was doing a lot of one-on-one coaching at that point, and also launching my first group coaching program. Over and over again, clients would say things like, "Heather, you've changed my life, and really helped me in my parenting." It was the soothing balm my soul was most craving.

The praise and validation felt amazing, but really it was more than that. I was doing exactly what I'd always yearned to do—help people—and doing it exactly how I'd always wanted to do it. As much as I'd loved going to therapy over the years, I'd never wanted to become a clinical therapist. Instead, I wanted to help people face their challenges and be able to ask them, "Okay, so what are you going to do about it?"

As a coach, I could drop f-bombs and be myself. I could call people on their bullshit excuses and help them see that the answers they'd been seeking elsewhere and from other people were usually best sourced from inside themselves. It felt so, so good being able to show up as myself, knowing that by doing so, I was making an even bigger impact on people's lives.

You could say that I was addicted to working, and I wouldn't argue with you, but my addiction was nuanced. Since grade school, I'd bought into the idea that had been projected onto me by teachers and school administrators that I was "too stupid" and "not cut out" to succeed. Now I had proof that they'd been wrong. I could not only succeed in my career and my life, but I could also do it on my own terms.

Allowing myself to feel like I was enough, to feel worthy, was incredibly healing. Finally, I could trust my gut and that little whisper inside me that had long suspected that I did have important gifts to offer the world. I mattered, my work mattered, and the healing that I felt from that was intense and life-changing.

I was addicted, sure, but not to work. I was healing at my core, learning to love and value myself. And it felt amazing.

Energized, Invigorated, and Numb

By Felix's first birthday, I would wake up, have a green juice, and get to work. The baby weight had come off so effortlessly that I'd basically abandoned exercise altogether. Working as much as I was also seemed like another reason that I was losing weight. "You look great!" people would exclaim, sometimes in tones of voice that conveyed surprise or, occasionally, jealousy. I wasn't especially concerned either way. I'd never had issues with my weight, which had always been in the healthy range.

Truth be told, my body had never ranked high on my priority list. My energy usually slumped as the day dragged on, but what else was new? It never occurred to me that I'd need more than a single serving of green juice to get through an active day. Having grown up in a household where food was more an obligation than an essential source of pleasure and well-being, I'd honestly never viewed food as necessary fuel. At dinnertime, I'd eat, but often that would be the first solid food I'd consumed all day.

Most of the time, I felt so revved up mentally and intellectually by the work I was doing that eating and paying attention to my body felt like a waste of time. I was serving others, helping them transform their lives and their parenting. Wasn't that fuel enough? While I felt good mentally, I was still ignoring my body's need for consistent nourishment. With time that would become an important growing edge for me.

Making the Break

As my mat leave approached its end, I knew that the time had come to quit my social work job, but actually doing it felt agonizing. The questions I'd been asking myself for some time continued to haunt me. How could I quit work that was so important for people who so badly needed me to act as their crusader? What kind of person could abandon a population that was *that* vulnerable? Overcome by guilt and shame, I finally did what I'd worked so hard to be able to do and submitted my official resignation. As much as I'd wanted this, making the final break felt torturous, even shameful. I was free, yes, and loving my work, but what would happen to my former social work clients? Who would help them, their children, and their children's children? It was a necessary but painful choice that would haunt me for years afterward.

A Weird Feeling

Lying on my bed pressing my hand firmly on my belly, I asked a friend to feel a bulge in my lower abdomen. "What is this?" I asked. She said she didn't know and told me to get it checked out. Figuring that my body was recovering from having Felix a year earlier, I once again convinced myself that my bulging abdomen and my ongoing fatigue were just a phase. Who isn't tired when breastfeeding and raising children, right?

In October, just weeks after quitting my social work job, I went to Las Vegas for my best friend's bachelorette weekend. Instead of feeling excited for a break from home and a new experience with my friend, I felt exhausted and not at all in the mindset to be surrounded by people I barely knew. But for my friend's sake, I went anyway.

During that weekend, I was happy to discover that one of the other bridesmaids was a dietician. I remember talking to her, telling her that my stomach felt weird even though I wasn't pregnant. I confessed how confused I still felt about food. What should I eat? Was breakfast really the most important meal? If so, what should I be having for breakfast? Years had passed since I'd been to that retreat in Asheville where I'd been introduced to "exotic" whole foods like avocados, but still it all felt like some distant planet I couldn't quite map out.

As the weeks rolled on, my abdominal bloat only increased. What had begun as the visual equivalent of early pregnancy, when only you can tell your mid-section is expanding, turned fairly quickly into something else entirely. As my overall body grew leaner, my middle increasingly protruded from underneath my shirt.

One day I was standing in the kitchen prepping a meal when I suddenly said to Bryan, "Wouldn't it be funny if I had cancer?" He looked at me, clearly not amused.

There was a conversation happening inside me that I didn't want to hear. It was almost like a dialogue between my mind and my body, and day by day, it grew a little louder and a little clearer. I did everything I could to drown it out, hoping I'd misheard, praying I was imagining it all. Maybe, just maybe, if I pretended not to hear, it would stop.

"I'm Not Pregnant"

By December, just a couple of months after going to Las Vegas, my abdomen had ballooned to the size of a late-term pregnancy. Yet I was also losing weight, and at an even faster rate. With each passing day, my body felt like a less hospitable place to be.

Eventually, I began experiencing night sweats that made for restless nights for me and Bryan both. We were exhausted and secretly worried, but every time Bryan insisted that I go to the hospital, I brushed him off. "I'm fine," I'd say nonchalantly. *It'll go away, won't it?* I'd think to myself, even though I intuitively knew that not to be true. As our sleepless nights and my constant complaining added up, Bryan grew increasingly frustrated.

Finally, at his urging, I went to a clinic near my house. I was annoyed about having to go, and adamant that I wouldn't spend hours waiting for a doctor who had no answers to give. They felt around my abdomen, which was undeniably hard, and asked if I was in any pain. When I said no, they told me to go the emergency room if that changed. *That's what any physician would say*, I remember thinking. I promptly left the clinic and returned home.

Days later, as my body began pushing even harder to get my attention, I went to the hospital, not at all happy about being there. Perhaps sensing this, or maybe because she was having a bad day herself, the nurse I saw that day did not take to me. In a clipped, irritated tone of voice, she said, "So you're here for mild back pain and bloating?" I could hear the patronizing judgment oozing from her every word. Assuming I'd be forced to wait for hours before seeing a doctor, I left and returned home instead of waiting to be seen. That afternoon, the hospital called me to follow up, which I believe they're obliged to do by law, but I didn't answer because I was at home sleeping.

The next day, as I was complaining to Bryan once again, he cut me off. "I'm driving you to the hospital, and we're not leaving until we see a doctor." A few hours later, when I checked into the hospital, the nurse looked at me, my abdomen visibly protruding from my shirt, and said, "You can go straight upstairs to OB. You don't have to check in down here."

"That's the point," I said. "I'm not pregnant."

Her energy, her comportment, and almost everything about her very suddenly changed. "Oh, okay," she said in a concerned tone of voice.

After they'd taken blood and a routine CT of my abdomen, a different nurse came to see us where we were waiting behind a privacy curtain. I'd had to hold off on eating because of the CT scan, so I was starving. "Honey," she said in a voice that was overly sweet, soft, and caring, "if you're hungry, your husband can go upstairs and get you a sub."

The second she left, I looked at Bryan, my heart thumping in my chest. "She knows something. This is bad."

He looked at me and nodded.

Crashing into Reality

I ate, and we waited. And waited.

The doctor finally opened the curtains after what felt like forever.

She was a tall, middle-aged woman. She looked directly at me. "Heather, it's not good. Based on your blood work and the CT, you have cancer. We just don't know what kind."

I will never forget that moment. Something I'd secretly known all along was being confirmed, as if my inner knowing was being validated. In that instant my insides met my outsides, and something inside me changed forever. It was the most visceral fear I'd ever felt.

You have cancer.

The C-word is loaded with so many stories and so much fear. I was sure that being sick meant that I was going to die. For the first time, I couldn't numb my fear or run away from it. I had no choice but to feel it, to be honest with myself and face my truth.

Felix was barely over a year old. Calvin had just turned four, and Logan was only eight. In that moment, the inner truth I'd tried so hard not to hear came crashing down, knocking down every ounce of reality I'd ever known and loved.

I had cancer. This was really happening. I couldn't avoid it now.

In the days that followed, I returned to the hospital to get a biopsy, and then to the doctor's office for the biopsy results. She diagnosed me with diffuse large B-cell lymphoma. Even with a diagnosis, however, I couldn't take immediate action. We were in the midst of the winter holidays and everything was delayed, including seeing an oncologist. It was traumatic holding information that terrifying and critical yet feeling utterly powerless to do anything about it.

I May Be Sick, but I'm Not a Liar

At the urging of a friend, I quickly scheduled an appointment at the top cancer treatment center in Detroit, Michigan, which is just across the border, less than an hour from where I live. The only thing I could control was getting a second opinion, so that's exactly what we would do.

Given how tight our financial situation had become, my friend generously offered to pay for my visit. Ashamed, but also desperate, I accepted her help. After having my medical test results forwarded to this new doctor, on the appointed date, my mom, my friend, and I drove to the appointment together. It was a literal life saver. Truthfully, if I didn't have the privileges that I have, I probably wouldn't have had access to that second opinion or that financial loan from a friend. Without both of those things, cancer probably would have killed me years ago.

"You have Burkitt's lymphoma, 100 percent. You were misdiagnosed," the doctor said almost as soon as he entered the room. "I'd like to do some tests to check your kidney function," he added, before asking to speak with me privately.

Once my friend and my mom had left the room, he asked if I'd ever been exposed to HIV through IV drug use or been with anyone who had HIV. I assured him that I had not, but he clearly didn't believe me. As I tried to reassure him that I was telling the truth, I immediately thought of John, Logan's father, whose intravenous drug use had always been prolific and varied. *I'll kill that fucker if he gave me some horrific disease,* I thought to myself.

At the end of the appointment, the doctor offered to reach out to the top oncologist in Windsor, where I lived. I thanked him, and as I was leaving, he asked his final questions. "How did you even get here? How are you able to get up and walk?" His voice sounded confused and almost disbelieving. I shrugged, unsure how to answer. I felt very, very sick. I *was* very, very sick. It had just never occurred to me that I had any option but to keep going.

Three Days Too Many

It was Logan's ninth birthday, and my dad was throwing him a laser tag birthday party. Too weak to join the celebration, I stayed home, heartbroken to be missing Logan's big day. I'd never imagined missing one of his birthday celebrations. It was a first, and not one I was proud of.

Mid-January in Southern Ontario is the start of months of biting cold that's often accompanied by snow and ice. In spite of the freezing temperatures outside, I was so hot I could hardly stand to exist in my own skin. I would open the nearest window, but even standing in front of it, I couldn't stop sweating.

"You have to go check yourself in today, Heather. You don't have until Tuesday," my mother-in-law, who was also a former oncology nurse, told me in a voice that was both fearful and matter-of-fact.

It was Saturday. On Tuesday I would meet with my new oncologist—I'll call her Dr. H. I wanted to wait, had assumed I would wait, but I could feel how sick I was, and how quickly I was getting sicker. Knowing my mother-in-law was right about my not having three more days, I agreed and went back to the emergency room, expecting to get some IV fluids to sustain me before returning home. From the ER, however, I was sent directly to oncology, where I was admitted, given a room, and told I'd begin chemo that night, before I'd ever even met Dr. H.

What's Happening?

Coming out of a deep sleep, not remembering what had happened to me in the last twelve hours, I was lying in a hospital bed surrounded by nurses, a few friends, and family. Just then the shock started to set in. My phone vibrated in my hand. I raised it to read my new text messages, but everything was blurry. I moved it around, trying to find the perfect angle where I could see a little bit of the light, but even then, only some words were legible.

I can hardly see. Is this normal?

Why was this happening to me? I'd expected to lose my hair immediately from chemo, but instead I lost the majority of my eyesight. Nearly blind, I could see people, but they were fuzzy, blurry colored blobs within vague outlines. Text, especially screen-sized, was much harder to make out.

Friends and family would call and text me, but in many more important ways I barely knew what was happening. One morning I'd woken up at home, and by that evening I was in the hospital undergoing chemotherapy. It was traumatic for all of us, but I often wonder if the trauma wasn't worse for Bryan and our boys. I was almost too sick to feel traumatized. Staying alive took what little energy I had left.

It Took a Village

With our finances so tight, Bryan kept working, which seemed like the right decision. We needed to maintain some level of stability and normalcy, if only for the kids.

Not that anything was normal, or that the kids were unaware of that fact. In my absence, my in-laws stepped in to help Bryan. The boys sometimes slept at home, and other times, at their grandparents' house. My children came and went from places according to schedules I was no longer a part of. For the first time in my life, I had to surrender to my village. For a period of time no one could define or predict, I would be unable to manage my schedule, my life, even my own children. Other people were deciding what to feed them, when to put them bed, and how much television they were allowed to watch.

My littlest, my baby, had just turned one. One milestone after another was occurring in my absence. I felt a deep, searing guilt that I couldn't shake. How could I be missing such a precious stage of his early development? What kind of mother did that make me? Logically, I knew I had no choice, but as most mothers know, logic doesn't often factor into how wholly we love our children or how deeply we yearn to nurture them, even when it exhausts us.

Some of my babies were bigger than others, but still… They were mine, but they were not with me, not around me, nowhere near my reach. Their absence pained me deeply, but my job now wasn't to care for them every day. My job was to survive. My job was to get through this so I wouldn't have to miss even more.

Meeting the Red Devil

As I got ready to shave my head, I blasted rap music in my hospital room. It was my way of turning what many might assume would be a sad, somber event into a celebratory one. This was no time for me to curl up, cry, and hide or worry about what other people thought. It was time to make noise. It was time to get loud and be a disruptor. Shaving my head didn't feel to me like giving up. It felt like taking control of what little I could.

"Can you get Carrie?" I asked Bryan as I was setting the mood for the raucous party I was envisioning in my mind. Carrie was already one of my favorite nurses; we'd connected almost immediately. She had a vibrant personality and a healthy sense of fun. *She* would get what I was doing. *She* would understand that this was no pity party.

The day before, a nurse had come into my room to start my chemo. Up to that point, the chemo bags had contained a clear liquid. This time, she'd brought a bag with red liquid, which the nurses referred to as the "red devil."

"This is the one that will make your hair fall out," the nurse had said as she started the drip.

I'd always loved and cared for my hair. My biggest fear now wasn't cutting it off. It was having it fall out in clumps. I didn't ever want to touch my scalp and come away with a handful of my own hair. Instead of waiting for the red devil to perform its deed, I'd asked Bryan to bring clippers to the hospital. I was ready to shave my head. I was just days into chemo, but somehow it already felt like time. And it would be a party—this party, to be exact.

"Do you want to do it?" I asked my mom, offering her the clippers as Bryan and Carrie looked on.

She hesitated. "No, not really... Do you want me to do it?" Her voice was shaky and filled with a dread that immediately grated on my nerves.

I wanted so badly for this to feel fun, to feel liberating, but the fact was, we were all raw, just in different ways. I was noticing that even the people who wanted to be there for me often couldn't do that when and how I needed them to. We were all suffering, but not in compatible ways at compatible times.

I handed her the clippers. First, she cut off my ponytail, which was matted after my having lain in a hospital bed for days on end. Once my hair was short enough, she began shaving the back of my head.

"Okay, that's good," she said a couple of minutes later.

Since my first round of chemo, my eyesight had begun to come back. I could see again, and more than anything I wanted to see myself without hair. I was connected at all times to an IV line, so I couldn't go far, but I did get up to look at myself in the mirror. There were patches all over my scalp. Irritated and completely unable to create space for my mother's experience or her emotions as she shaved her twenty-seven-year-old daughter's head between bouts of chemo, I grabbed the clippers.

After finishing the job myself, I looked in the mirror one more time. For months, as my health had declined, my hair had grown brittle and lackluster, which had been frustrating. After so many years of caring for and styling my long hair, I'd secretly been dreaming about shaving my head. And now, I'd done it.

Looking at myself, I felt a rush of intense emotion. *You did it, Heather. You really fucking did it.* In that instant, almost all of my accomplishments—getting my university degree, landing my social work job, growing my coaching business, even being a teen mom—paled in comparison. I was undergoing chemo, and I'd just shaved my head. It felt amazing. At long last, after all these years, I finally felt proud of myself.

End of Chapter Exercise: Want, Crave, Desire

Around the time of my diagnosis, I'd begun using Danielle LaPorte's *Desire Map*. In that book, LaPorte explains that our accomplishments only matter to us because of how they make us feel. Essentially, we don't yearn to accomplish our goals for their own sake; we're motivated to accomplish a task or achieve a goal because of the feeling we think it's going to give us. Therefore, rather than focusing on goals, we should focus on what we most desire to feel.

To understand our desires, she says, we first need to understand how we want to feel, which she calls our Core Desired Feelings, or CDFs. Once we know those, we're free to identify and pursue activities, alliances, and outcomes that align with our CDFs.

When the "red devil" arrived and I was faced with needing to shave my head, I remember thinking about how I wanted the experience to feel and deciding, *I'm not going to be a victim here. I'm going to consciously shift how I feel.* That allowed me to regain some sense of control and assume responsibility for my mental and emotional health. Obviously, I didn't know what the future held for me, but I could control my experience of the present. It was transformational and a huge reason that I was able, from that point forward, to show up for my healing journey in the ways that I did.

Since then, I've developed a simpler way for my clients to identify how they want to feel. I call it making your "Want/Crave/Desire" list. This list is always a work in progress, and something you can and should change as your clarity increases. It's also an immensely valuable way of focusing on activities, pursuits, and alliances that support how you want to feel, in good times and in tough times.

To begin your list, carve out fifteen or twenty minutes of uninterrupted quiet time. Take out your notebook, and at the top of the page write three separate column headers:

I want...	I crave...	I desire...

In each column, write whatever comes to mind—without worrying about how you're defining each category. Let your intuition lead the way and write what *feels right to you* in each column. There are no right or wrong answers here, and nothing is too small, big, or contradictory to put on your list. It's perfectly normal to desire solitude and connection or to crave fulfillment and desire fewer to-dos. All that matters is that your list is a true reflection of *you* and *your* wants, cravings, and desires, not what you feel you *should* want, crave, and desire.

Once you're done filling these three columns, take a few minutes to sit with the *feeling* that you think achieving each want, craving, and desire will give you, then write those feelings down beside the acts you've chosen to achieve them.

For example, I played music and surrounded myself with people I love while I shaved my head because I wanted to have fun and feel joy; I wanted to make it a positive experience. Even though I was uncomfortable, scared, and sad, I chose to change the environment to bring it more in alignment with how I wanted to feel. That allowed me to have a mostly positive experience. In order to achieve those feelings, I had to first actively choose how I wanted to feel and then change my energy and my surroundings to support them. It's an intentional way of aligning your desired feelings with what you do every day.

7

Angels All Around Us

"**OKAY, YOU'VE FINALLY** got my attention."

I'd spoken those words a few weeks earlier while standing in front of the hospital, just after learning that I did in fact have cancer. I'd been looking up at the sky when I said them, speaking to some spiritual being or force I'd never consciously acknowledged believing in.

During the weeks that had passed since that moment, a lot more than my hair had changed. I was now peeing out what looked like Pepto-Bismol. It was a thick bright pink liquid that seemed to come out of me by the pint all day, every day.

The Pepto-Bismol, I soon learned, was in fact the skin cells from dead tumors. Thanks to chemotherapy, the cancer cells were pouring out of me at a rate that felt exhausting, mostly because they needed to escape my body so often. Weak and depleted, I dragged my body, as well as the IV line that was now attached to me 24/7, to the bathroom over and over again. The trip often felt like several journeys too many, but the cancer cells were leaving me, so whenever the urge to pee arose, I got up.

In so many ways and on so many levels, I was purging; but it was more than that, really. I was transforming, and nowhere so fully as deep inside myself, on a spiritual level I hadn't previously dared to access.

Meeting Batman

"You did it," she said, her voice upbeat and also a little surprised.

"I've heard really good things about you," I offered, feeling weak and tired, but also relieved to have her there, in my room, by my side.

It was pitch black outside when I first met Dr. H, aka Batman, who, it turns out, is a tiny but mighty woman with blond hair. She had a clean-cut, sophisticated appearance and the authoritative, no-nonsense manner of a hardworking doctor who regularly deals in matters of life and death. Without noise or warning, her figure had appeared at my bedside. She'd come to check my vitals.

"Heather," she continued, "we didn't know how your body would respond to the chemo. We had to move very quickly when you got here. But your body is responding, which means the cancer is rapidly growing, which is great because chemo reacts well to live cancer cells. We didn't know what was going to happen, but your body seems to be reacting well."

I was too exhausted to feel stressed, but her words still felt like a soothing balm. If peeing out Pepto-Bismol was what healing required, I'd take it. My cancer, which was in fact Burkitt's lymphoma, wasn't just advanced. It was stage four Burkitt's lymphoma—as in, the final stage. My mother-in-law, a former oncology nurse, had been correct when she'd said I didn't have any time to spare. I really was *that* sick. Every hour, every day prior to this one, the tumors inside my abdomen had been aggressively stealing my life, hoarding what little hope there was left.

The Burden (and Relief) of Knowing

They say knowledge is power. I believe that's true, but when you're staring down late stage cancer that really could, and really would, take your life and deprive your three young children of their mother, ignorance can start to sound like bliss.

There was a part of me that wanted Batman to come save the day (as in, my life) without my having to know why I needed her. I was scared, really scared, and sorely missing my family and my life. At the same time, though, cancer was opening up doors inside and around me that I'd never known I could access.

Word about my cancer and chemo had spread fast. Soon after being admitted to oncology, I began getting phone calls, text messages, and emails. People wanted to know what was happening, how I was feeling, and what I needed. Two friends organized fundraisers—one online and another an in-person event. People I'd never even met were going out of their way to help and support me. My life was on the line, yes, but all was not lost. I could stay in my hospital bed, knowing that entire groups of people were working hard to protect and preserve my and my family's health and well-being.

You have a community, Heather. Look at what they're doing for you. You don't have to feel alone anymore. You never were alone.

I'd never felt as supported and cared for as I did then.

There would be many challenges ahead, but now there were people, and even more were popping out of the woodwork, mobilizing, organizing, assisting, and donating on my behalf every day. The experience was eye-opening, and its effects, long-lasting. Never again would I turn a blind eye to my own and others' fundamental need for community. Creating community, especially among women, would eventually become a central part of my life's purpose and my life's work. I have cancer—and the many incredible souls who jumped at the chance to help me—to thank for that.

Full-Body Rejection

Of course, it wasn't all sunshine and rainbows. Foul substances were coming out of both ends—as in, I was simultaneously vomiting and shitting the bed—when this firefighter-turned-nurse entered my room. Humiliated but unable to control the oral and rectal emissions that were forcing their way out of me, I did what any woman in such a vulnerable position would do.

"I'm usually a lot cuter than this, I swear!" I announced to him, trying to sound confident and upbeat before leaning, once again, into my vomit bowl as my bowels rejected whatever air, water, or food they couldn't handle now that I was undergoing chemo.

I don't think he was entirely convinced, but he did smile, or so I like to tell myself. A girl can dream, right? When your body is literally dying, and when the treatment you're doing to save it is making you puke, shit your bed, piss Pepto-Bismol, and generally turn into a bald, skinny blob you hardly recognize, you have to hold on to whatever hope you can. In those moments, and the many months that followed, little bursts of hope, irreverence, spunk, spirit, and inappropriate humor can save you, as they did me, many times.

My abdomen shrank fast in the first few days of chemo, and alongside it my middle morphed into the post-tumor version of a new mother's belly—encircled by folds of excess skin it no longer needed but couldn't immediately shed. My tumors were shrinking, but my body still felt like someone else's. Lying in bed day after day, often too weak to stand, my muscles atrophied quickly. I had little strength or stamina, and my stomach hurt constantly.

A week or so after first meeting the red devil and shaving my head, I'd begun to feel frustrated; what little hair I had left still wasn't falling out. *Did I go bald for nothing?* I'd wondered more than once, feeling vaguely pissed off. Soon afterward, however, I got my answer. One day I rubbed my head, and all the peach fuzz I had left came right off. Along with it went my pubes, so at no extra charge, the hospital gave me the equivalent of a Brazilian wax that lasted for months.

My appetite was often low to non-existent; most of the time, food had no appeal. The rare times when my appetite did return, I felt like a drug addict dying for a quick hit. *Food! Give me food! I'm starving!* My hunger arrived in intense bursts, each one filled with cravings that make pregnancy cravings seem comparatively meek.

Over and over again, the hospital dietician told me to order McDonald's because I "needed the calories." But I wanted real food, whole food, food that could actually nourish and help to heal my body. Against the hospital's advice, I asked a local café to make me smoothies and other fresh, wholesome food that my family would then deliver to me. It was strictly advised against; fruits and vegetables, the hospital explained, could have live bacteria that could make an immune-compromised person like myself very sick.

"Can you explain to me how McDonald's is going to nourish my body?" I'd ask.

Clearly uncomfortable with my questions, the hospital dietician gave me clipped, incomplete explanations that emphasized calories and avoided any mention of actual nutrients. Well aware that there was a lot I needed to learn about food, I was sincerely interested in knowing more, but entirely unconvinced that chemical-laden fast food was the answer.

Every time she'd begin her McDonald's pitch, I'd nod politely, and then I'd take another sip of my smoothie or bite of my veggie-packed salad or sandwich, usually while looking directly at her, and making sure to smile as kindly as I could.

My inner rebel was alive and well and growing stronger by the day.

Since I wouldn't eat the McDonald's they'd prescribed, every day I'd get a shot glass of an extremely intense, dense version of Ensure.

"You *have to* drink this, Heather," one nurse after another would tell me.

"Your body needs the calories to heal, Heather," the dietician would add.

"I physically can't," I'd explain. "It makes me gag. I'll vomit it right up."

I didn't drink it. I literally couldn't. Instead, I ate whatever food appealed to me whenever my body would let me eat it.

To be honest, though, vomiting wasn't always a deterrent. One day during one of my *feed me now* moments, I had my sister bring me chicken parmesan from a local pizza place called Franco's. To this day, my sister still talks about how fast I ate every last bite of food on that plate.

"Slow down," she kept telling me.

The food tasted so, so good.

"You're going to puke," she said.

"I don't care!" I exclaimed, literally shoving one bite after another into my mouth.

Moments later, as if on cue, I did what we both knew I would do and promptly vomited every bite I'd eaten.

"That was so good," I said to her once the entire meal had left my body.

"What? You didn't even take in the calories!" she said.

"I know, but going in, it tasted *soooooo* amazing. It was so worth it."

I was never so grateful for food as I was during my months in chemo. Having an appetite felt like this incredible gift, and every bite like an orgasm in my mouth.

What I Have Is Not Who I Am

I would feel so, so sick, but then I'd get on a coaching call with a client and my entire body would start to buzz. It was a weird but also healing experience, as if coaching lit me up so wholly that my body could repair itself just enough to sustain me through my client calls.

I'm sure people worried about me, still working from my hospital bed. Conventional thinking was that I was sick, that I needed to focus on resting in order to heal. Those thoughts had crossed my mind, too, especially during my first days in the hospital. Very quickly, though, I realized that healing is a highly personalized process; we all do it differently. Continuing to coach clients, I realized, was more than a financial necessity. For me it was also an important part of my healing process.

Being of service to others had always been essential to my feeling alive. To disconnect from my purpose—my coaching work—would have been a way of dying, not healing. Instead of pausing my coaching business, I called my clients soon after my first round of chemo to let them know what was happening. "If I'm too sick to work with you, I'll let you know, but if I'm not, I'll show up for you," I told each of them. There were indeed times when I was too sick to show up. When that happened, I'd reschedule. Every time I was able to coach, though, I'd feel that buzzing sensation. As often as possible, I tried to make my healing work around my coaching. It fueled me like little else could.

Learning to Receive

While I was primarily focused on healing, our growing need for money was never far from my mind. Despite knowing that I had to continue working, even during chemo, when Bryan and I learned how much had been raised from the two fundraisers, we were tempted not to take the money. It was money we desperately needed, but still—fourteen thousand dollars was a lot more than we'd ever imagined receiving.

Both the online and in-person fundraising events had been big successes. For the in-person fundraising event, two competing companies—the car dealership Bryan worked for at the time, and its direct competitor—had united to sponsor the event. Online and offline, people had donated money and prizes, bought tickets, and spread the word to friends, family, and neighbors. It was beyond heartwarming, and we both felt enormously grateful. All of these people, even entire companies, had rallied around our family. They'd made a point of showing us that they cared, and they'd done it by collecting funds that we sorely needed to survive.

Still, though, just the idea of taking that money felt deeply uncomfortable. After so many years of doing whatever I had to in order to survive on my own, an entire community was now showing up to let us know we mattered. People had spent weeks organizing and arranging these events. The energy and the money felt like a lot to just receive. How would we ever repay that kind of debt of gratitude?

At the same time, we knew the money would allow us to pay bills we were struggling to pay. It was also significant in other ways that took me a little longer to see. My friends who'd organized the fundraisers had called me during the planning stages, getting my okay or input on various details. During our calls, I'd found myself helping them process their grief over my cancer. We were friends, but during that time I was acting as their coach too. They were resisting feeling the fear, worry, and other emotions my illness was creating. I understood their struggle. I was navigating it, too, although on a different level.

What I eventually came to understand was that the fundraisers and the energy they'd generated for them were also part of *their* healing process. Not accepting the money they raised would be unfair and insensitive to them.

It was a lesson I needed to learn at the time—when we reject opportunities to receive, we rob ourselves and others of profound growth and connection. The Universe operates on a model of giving and receiving. In order to participate in the Universe's natural tendency toward abundance, we have to do both.

Receiving that money ultimately became another powerful lesson in building community—that in order to create community as a healer, you have to learn to receive healing too.

Energy Conservation

As my physical, spiritual, and emotional energy, as well as my ability to eat, walk, and stay awake waxed and waned from one chemo treatment to the next, I became hyperaware of my energy stores. What was giving me energy? What was depleting my energy? I needed every last ounce I could find.

Since childhood, I'd always been sensitive to people's energy, noise levels, even smells. To this day, all of it can have a big impact on me. What I began to realize during cancer treatment was how different people and environments were impacting me. I was a giver, yes, and a coach and leader by nature, but there were limits to how much I could give, and how often I did.

The deeper I got into chemo, the more I began to respect my energy boundaries. There were days and times when I couldn't manage certain people's needs, and other times when I could. This didn't apply to coaching, which I loved from start to finish. However, throughout the rest of my life, I was noticing how I felt when I hung up from phone calls, logged on to social media, or interacted with one nurse versus another. The people, places, and things I surrounded myself with impacted my energy, and for the first time in my life, I wasn't just seeing that, I was doing something about it.

When a nurse was cranky, I'd try to seek out nicer ones, or at least find out when they'd be on duty next. I loved Dr. H, but some of the other doctors were assholes. I couldn't avoid them, but I didn't prolong their stay by oversharing either. I'd answer their questions, but without elaborating, and quietly rejoice the moment they left my room. With friends and family, on days when I felt off or like I couldn't give what they seemed to want from me, I'd say that I was too tired to talk.

I sincerely appreciated how much people were doing for us, but I had to focus on my one and only goal—surviving. Setting boundaries and prioritizing my energy was a non-negotiable part of that healing. I also needed as much energy as possible for my children, even if, at this particular moment in time, I wasn't able to spend as much time with them as usual.

My Mom Is Sick, but She's Still My Mom

"OMG, I'm going to die! It smells *so* bad in here!" Logan would scream, holding his hands over his nose and mouth as he jumped up to escape.

To this day, he insists that my chemo farts were the worst smell he's ever encountered. The worst part was, I couldn't always tell. My stomach was in perpetual turmoil, my body was off-gassing toxic fumes, and my oldest child was left to suffer the consequences.

Calvin and Felix were still too young, but at nine years old, Logan could occasionally sleep over at the hospital. Each time, we'd arrange it in advance so the hospital facility staff could reserve a cot and roll it into my room on the appointed day. I don't remember having a television in my hospital room, but we did usually watch a movie on a device of some kind.

However, the true highlight of each visit was always morning time. Logan loved the café in the hospital lobby. Every time he'd sleep at the hospital, I'd muster all of my energy and courage to make the trip. It was a Herculean effort, getting out of bed, walking to the elevator, and dragging my IV line with me all the way downstairs. We'd get him hot chocolate and a donut, or whatever he wanted, and then make the long trek back to my room.

That trip felt incredibly taxing, but he was nine, and he needed his mom. He pushed me to show up for him, so I did. It was grueling at moments when my energy was especially low or my pain, extra gruesome. It didn't feel easy, but by letting him push me to do a little more than I thought I could, I was able to be the leader of my own healing process. Just by expecting me to be there for him, Logan helped me to see that. Just by letting me know he still needed me, he forced me to make that extra effort to heal a little more, a little faster, than I felt I could.

Healing at Home

Between rounds of chemo, I would return home to rest, usually for a couple of weeks at a time. It was a weird feeling, floating in and out of my own home, life, and family. It wasn't as if I hadn't seen them, of course. In addition to Logan's periodic hospital sleepovers, Bryan would stop by the hospital after work most days. I appreciated the gesture, but I also felt frustrated by how tired he always was. I'd plead with him to take better care of himself, all too aware of how he'd been emotionally depleted by the trauma we were all living through. His face would glaze over, almost as soon as I began talking. *I can't take in anymore* was written all over his face. He was sitting next to my bed, but he couldn't hear me. He was surviving, but just barely. He wasn't the only adult in my family who was reacting that way.

Even with cancer, even while I was undergoing chemo, everyone still needed me, maybe even more than ever. They needed to connect with me, and they needed my reassurance that I'd be okay. Over and over again, they came to me to find out how to control their big emotions. It made me angry—sometimes, really angry. I desperately needed all of the adults in my family to show up, but some of them couldn't do that because they didn't know how to take care of themselves. Seeing that and remembering what it felt like to be needed at that level from my sickbed, even now I can get triggered when people talk about it being "selfish" to take care of themselves. If your loved one gets sick, is it selfish for you to neglect yourself so much that you barely have the energy to show up for them in their hours of need?

The tension was real; the dynamic, hard to navigate. The fact was, we were all charting new territory. None of us knew what lay ahead. Our different reactions to the situation weren't anyone's fault, but it was hard connecting, even during a time when we all really needed to.

People want to believe that something like cancer would bring friends and family together. It can do that, at times, but healing, like life, is anything but perfect. Sometimes it really hurts, and in more ways than you feel able to handle.

On weekends, Bryan would sometimes bring all three boys to the hospital, but that wasn't easy either. They were young and their mother was in a hospital bed with cancer. It was a lot to take in, and most often, they'd start to fight, sometimes loudly. I was too tired and happy to see them to worry about their behavior—they could have spit in my face, and I'd barely have noticed—but their constant bickering stressed Bryan out. He'd reprimand them, which then frustrated me. Oftentimes, they'd leave fairly soon after arriving.

The experience wore on all of us.

When I was home between rounds of chemo, my energy would ebb and flow. I remember lying in bed, knowing that I could stay there, watching television, doing nothing. No one would question me. No one would ask me to do anything. I was healing from my last round of chemo and preparing my body for the next round.

But I was determined to live, and I was all too aware that sleep has always been my drug of choice, so as often as I could, I pushed myself to get up. On a visceral level I knew that choosing to live couldn't just be something I told myself I was doing or would do later. It had to be something I was actively pursuing—in real time, in the here and now, even when it felt really, really challenging.

If I wanted to build my business, that meant spending time working on my business. Even when I didn't feel up to it, I'd drag my laptop into bed with me and do research, schedule client calls, or reply to emails. I had to be a mom, too, whenever I could. At one point, Logan began acting out. When I approached him about the choices he'd been making, we talked about how he was feeling. During that conversation, he confessed to me that he wanted to get his ear pierced. Knowing that he was in pain and yearning to do something—anything— to take control of his pain, I agreed to take him. I hated the idea of him having a pierced ear. However, he needed this, and

I could be a part of his healing by helping him do it, so with my head still very bald, I put on lipstick and off we went to the mall.

Even on my good days, however, there were limits to what I could manage and when. In addition to my nausea and noxious farting, the chemo caused excruciating bone pain. To cope with the agony, my entire body would sometimes shake violently and involuntarily. In those moments, the pain was so all-consuming that I wasn't aware who was even in the room with me. To this day, I don't know if my children ever saw me during one of my shaking episodes, but even now, whenever they see me in bed, they reflexively ask me if I'm okay. Mom being in bed, even all these years later, remains a scary thing.

Shitting the Bed

After weeks of going into and out of chemo, I began to feel this incredible freedom. I could look however I wanted, say whatever I wanted, be whoever I wanted. No one would judge me. I still had cancer, and, yes, I was undergoing chemo. Again. Somehow, though, I felt like a lot of the responsibility I'd always carried around was being lifted off my plate. I could finally breathe deeply again. I had a newfound feeling of space and freedom with no strings attached—except death, of course.

My fear of dying, of leaving my family behind, still tugged at me. The idea of leaving three young sons behind was so terrifying, it was almost surreal. *How is this even happening to me?* I'd ask myself sometimes, trying to make sense of my altered reality.

Cycling between these many thoughts and emotions, one night I woke up in my hospital bed. It was pitch black outside, my body was in agony, and I was once again vomiting while shitting the bed. I didn't just think I was dying this time; I also felt like I was.

It was humbling, feeling that vulnerable and powerless, but I also knew there was nothing else anyone could do for me. I had to accept what was happening, to surrender to it and feel it all. I couldn't move, and my pain and physical discomfort were too extreme to even call a nurse. I had no choice but to be cracked open, which I let happen willingly. On a deep level, I sensed that this wasn't a time to react or even feel afraid. This was a time to be still, to accept, and to receive.

Just then, a warm feeling overcame me, and in spite of what my body was doing, I felt safe. There was white light all around me and I knew that while I was the only person in my room, I wasn't actually alone. There were angels around me, each one emitting light, all of them taking turns by my side. They were flowing toward me, one by one, like a river of love and support. I knew right then that I was being protected, that I wasn't alone and never had been.

On the left side of me, by my heart, I suddenly felt this weird plucking feeling, as if the white light—the stream of angels coming to my side—were taking old limiting beliefs out of me and replacing them with healing ones. In that moment I didn't quite know what was being plucked away or put in, only that it was a form of healing. These were sacred gifts that I could only receive if I was willing to let go and be plucked in order to get better and live.

The next morning, after months of feeling terrified that I'd die and leave my family so soon, I woke up with a new and surprising realization:

I'm going to be okay.

I'm going to live.

I'd reached the rock bottom of my suffering. It was behind me now. I had made it.

I'm going to be okay.

This new understanding rang through me, like a clear bell I'd been longing to hear. Finally, at long last, it was time to start living—*really* living—and begin honoring myself, my worth, and all of my big hopes and dreams.

8

Relearning How to Live

MY VISIT WITH ANGELS was a profoundly pivotal experience and the start of my learning what it felt like to truly live. However, it wasn't the only life-changing moment in my healing journey. There had been others—moments when I'd felt my fear at such a visceral level, I'd been forced to measure the strength of my most primal fears against my desire to live.

One of these other moments had also occurred at night, in between rounds of chemo, while lying on my bathroom floor at home, feeling sick and depleted. Yet again, words had echoed inside me, haunting me on every imaginable level.

You're dying, Heather.

You're a twenty-eight-year-old mother of three boys, and you're dying.

Practically kissing the floor, too worried about inconveniencing my family to wake them up, I barely had the strength to get up when I had a sudden realization.

But Heather, you're not dead yet.

That moment, too, had changed me on a deep and lasting level. It was suddenly clear—I wasn't afraid of dying; I'd just never known what it felt like to live. And just like that, I embarked on a quest, determined to learn what I needed to learn in order to fight for my life every single day. Fear would come up at times, but I no longer needed to live from a place of fear. Worrying about living up to other people's expectations, being judged as a "not good enough" mother, not parenting the "right" way, or failing in my business—these were all fears I was shedding, little by little, day by day. I could finally focus on what I desired, rather than what I wanted to get rid of.

Equipped with this new sense of purpose, I walked out of the hospital, bald, skinny, and weak, but also free. It was April, and after four rounds of chemo in less than five months, I'd been cleared to go live my life.

Asking New Questions

What does it mean to feel fully alive—in your body and your life? What does it mean to be brave and show up even when you're scared? Who do you want to be, Heather? What do you want to do?

Questions like these went through my mind, day in and day out.

The message I'd asked for from the Universe when I'd looked up at the sky months earlier and said I was listening had finally come through loud and clear. If I wanted to keep my life, I would have to claim it. I had angels, yes, but I also needed to proactively participate in the act of living. It wouldn't be all puffy clouds and loving embraces. This was a real opportunity to co-create the life I desired, and it wasn't going to be easy.

This message was one I literally couldn't hear often enough, a drumbeat I had on endless replay in my mind, if only to convince my fearful lizard brain that I was, in fact, capable of this monumental feat known as living, that I could develop the grit it would demand of me. Finally, I would have to learn how to live *my* life on *my* terms as *my*self.

But what did that really mean? What would that look and feel like?

Even asking these questions felt terrifying. After all, living would mean chasing my big dreams and continually failing on my way toward success. It would mean showing up again and again, even when everything felt hard. It would also mean being myself and sometimes getting rejected. To truly live, I would have to start facing my feelings of unworthiness and allowing myself to be vulnerable. If ever there was a time to be brave, surely it was now.

Home Alone

Making a simple, nutritious dinner took every ounce of energy I had, but making that effort felt important. My body needed nourishment and my children needed nurturing *and* nourishment. Each step of the cooking process felt impossibly taxing, but I persevered, determined to serve a balanced meal. Finally done, I'd serve the food and collapse into a chair to eat. Moments later, most of the food I'd made would be scraped into the garbage. In my absence, my children had adapted, developing new routines and habits that included a preference for processed convenience food. My healthy dinners were an unwelcome disruption from what had become their "new normal."

I was hugely relieved to be back home where I belonged, but the transition wasn't seamless. In weird ways I was an outsider, and still the "sick one" in the house. My energy came and went, and physically I was fragile, still in a lot of pain, and vomiting often.

At the same time, I felt invigorated on a level I hadn't been in a long time, if ever. Even on my bad days the fact was, I'd survived. I was officially cancer-free. This was my big opportunity and I was determined not to waste it. *You can do anything, Heather! Go for it! You're* alive*!*

Yet also, I already had a life, and in that sense, an already full plate with a family that had found their way during my absence. I was free, but only sort of. It was an exciting but also strange and awkward time. There were suddenly no nurses or doctors checking on me and very few appointments I needed to keep. With the boys in school and Bryan working, I was often home alone, forever facing that same void inside myself and my life.

What do you want to do with your life, Heather? Who do you want to be?

Taking Courageous Action

"I need to get stronger," I announced. "I just finished chemo, so I've lost all of my strength. I want my stamina back."

Still mostly bald and devoid of all muscle, I'd walked into a local gym. The trainer I was speaking with focused on something called "strength training," which meant nothing to me at the time. I'd never been a gym girl.

My new trainer seemed to believe in building strength and fitness in a healthy, gradual way. That seemed like a good sign, but still, I was the proverbial fish out of water. However, doing hard and uncomfortable things needed to become my new norm, and my health, my number-one, non-negotiable priority. I wanted to feel like the body I was inhabiting was actually mine again. And more than anything, I wanted to feel good. I yearned to feel alive, to feel sensations that were far removed from pain and death. I wanted to look around and feel proud of myself for taking ownership of myself, my health, and my life.

Exercise, like healthy eating, meditation, and other mindfulness practices, had been one of my many health and wellness Band-Aids, useful and relevant when I "needed" it. Over the years, I'd gone on periodic kicks, getting into yoga or running for a period of days or weeks. As soon as I felt better, I'd tell myself I was "good," meaning that I could skip it again. Inevitably, time would pass, my anxiety would again increase to an intolerable level, and I'd go on another yoga, running, or walking kick.

Prior to cancer, exercising regularly to maintain optimal health and prevent my anxiety levels from spiking had never even occurred to me. Now that I knew what poor health felt like and how much was actually at stake when I ignored it, I could see that everything I'd ever yearned for was on the other side of health and the habits that would support it. My mental/emotional resistance, whether to the gym, cooking nutritious food, or practicing mindfulness consistently, no longer mattered. Making new and healthier choices was a very real "now or never" opportunity.

A Living, Breathing Roadblock

Mentally, I was more than ready to jump back into my normal life, but my body could only manage baby steps. Reconciling the discrepancies between them was a steep learning curve. I would show up—to the gym, as a mother, or in my capacity as a business owner—only to be reminded that my body needed to have its say. *You're going to vomit. Oh, and here's more bone pain too.*

That struggle between my mind and body, which had intensified during chemo, only worsened now that I was cancer-free. Would I have to wait forever? How much more time would my body need to heal? This was the first time in my life I'd listened to my body. It was telling me to be patient, to let it heal at its own pace; but mentally, I was revving and ready to roar, forever frustrated by the limitations imposed on me by my body.

As much as I yearned to resume my normal life, I still needed extra support. My mother-in-law, a former oncology nurse who had been my home nurse during chemo when I'd needed daily injections, still came over to cook and clean. It was a blessing in so many ways. The children were very attentive to her, and I appreciated how consistent she was, feeding them regular meals and ensuring that they were on a schedule. It was also difficult, though. My home didn't entirely feel like my own, and even my children weren't always available to me. Sometimes I'd wake up from a nap, excited to do something fun with them, only to find out that their schedule didn't allow for that.

I was sincerely grateful for all the help we had gotten and were still getting, as well as everyone who had gone so far out of their way to help us. At the same time, I wanted my life back so fucking badly. Would my body ever let me have it?

Being with the Pain

My impatience occasionally turned to anger, but always my body would win. Vomiting had become so commonplace, it barely bothered me anymore, but my bone pain was too excruciating to ignore. However, it did have one upside: Percocet.

Anyone who tells you they don't like pain meds is lying, or so I might have said back then. Each prescription pain pill felt amazing—really, seriously amazing—going in like a numbing rush, taking away everything I didn't want and leaving me in a state of pain-free bliss. Within a few hours, however, the effects would wear off, the pain would edge back, and I'd get gut rot. More often than not, my body would also be overcome by fatigue, as if my limbs were suddenly many times their actual weight. For a period of time, I would become a living, breathing dead weight in my bed, barely able to move a finger, much less an arm or leg.

Even all these months after chemo, with my bone pain still occurring regularly, I kept getting Percocet prescriptions. I was taking the pills, but also increasingly worried about taking them. *Shouldn't I be off these by now?* Wanting to wean myself off them, I went from taking two at a time down to taking one. But I always made sure not to tell Bryan when I did take one.

I wasn't just still taking my pain meds. I was hiding them too.

More often than I wanted anyone to know, I would sneak into the kitchen, making sure no one was watching, and open the cupboard and place a pill in my mouth. Each time, I had to decide—did I want to numb the pain or feel the pain? It wasn't always a tough choice. Pain is physically and emotionally draining. Feeling the absence of pain was seductive, and here was Percocet, ready and able to take away my pain.

At the same time, though, I knew I was becoming addicted to the numbing relief that each pill provided. Without fail, once the soothing effect wore off, I would feel like shit, knowing that I was hiding, favoring numbness over truth. I was failing to be as brave as I'd wanted to become, sacrificing myself in order to avoid the deep discomfort my body was experiencing.

Fortunately, my memories of John, Logan's chronically addicted father, returned to show me what I needed to do. For Logan's sake, I couldn't risk addiction. I had to find a way to be with the pain, to get through it without pharmaceuticals, even though the pain really was *that* bad.

Reconciling with New Priorities

While I often faced tough choices, in many ways my life was a blank canvas; I could create whatever I chose. Every new day was a gift, and I knew it.

Near the end of my chemo treatments, Dr. H had told me that if I was going to relapse, it would probably happen within the first ten months after chemo. I tried not to dwell on that fact, but at all times there was a clock ticking in my subconscious.

Determined not just to survive my first ten months, but also to heal so I could live a full and vibrant life from that point onward, I continued to research natural health therapies. I had no regrets about undergoing chemo—it had saved my life—but I also had very real questions about how much traditional medicine could do for me at this stage in my journey.

Months earlier, I'd met with an oncology naturopathic doctor named Dr. Meighan Valero. She offered the vitamin C injection therapy that I knew I wanted. My medical doctors had advised against my getting them during chemo, but now done with chemo, I was free to begin.

Dr. Valero felt it was important for me to get vitamin C injections consistently for a period of months. The vitamin is injected in such high quantities that once it enters the body, it transforms from an antioxidant into an oxidative treatment, which, similar to chemo, causes selective cytotoxicity. In other words, it causes cancer cells to die.

Meeting with Dr. Valero post-chemo, I was reminded how much I trusted her. She had stayed in touch with Dr. H and followed my medical treatments and was now prepared to dial my care into my precise needs at any given time. Working with her didn't just feel right; it felt mandatory. At the core of my being, I believed that I'd survive and heal if I followed Dr. Valero's guidance. I was trusting my gut, investing in my intuitive knowing that working with her was a vital part of my healing journey.

However, this was an alternative therapy, so the cost would be out of pocket. Once again, we didn't have that money at our disposal. While Bryan was fully supportive of my desire to work with Dr. Valero, other family members, as well as some friends, didn't hesitate to tell me that they thought that alternative health was nonsense; that I was wasting money we badly needed to support ourselves.

I agonized about the decision but eventually realized that I had to trust myself and my values, not give in to the woman other people wanted me to be. Getting the injections felt like the right next step. However, in order to work with Dr. Valero, we would have to sell our camping trailer. Was I really willing to take away my children's vacations to get vitamin C injections? What kind of mother would do that?

Heather, right now you can give them a mother, or you can give them vacations.

My choice came with a heavy load of guilt, but we sold the RV, and off I went to Dr. Valero's office, twice a week for an entire year. Sacrificing one summer's vacations would allow us to enjoy years of fun, connection, and, yes, plenty of vacation travel together.

When I arrived for one of my first vitamin C treatments, I told Dr. Valero that I was here to stay, that I'd be around for my kids. She remembers being impressed by my certainty, especially after having had stage four cancer so recently.

Dr. Valero also knew that I'd come closer to dying than even I realized. The Pepto-Bismol–like solution that had come out of me during chemo had been a symptom of tumor lysis syndrome, a potentially fatal condition that can occur when large numbers of cancer cells are killed very quickly. When that happens, those cells can get released into the bloodstream, and levels of uric acid, potassium, and phosphorus can rise faster than the kidneys are capable of removing them. Even if cancer hadn't killed me, tumor lysis syndrome easily could have.

A Place of Empowerment

Dr. Valero's office was sparse back then, with one chair, a tiny refrigerator, a large screen television, and a perpetually sanitized but makeshift Ikea countertop where she'd mix up the bags for my treatments. It was a sharp contrast to the busy but serene spa-like office she maintains today.

Empty or not, her office was a place of hope for me. I felt empowered there. She was committed to me and my health, and I trusted her with my life. Her patients were also interesting, sometimes recommending books about alternative healing and health.

Years later I would learn that Dr. Valero was living with friends during our first months working together, healing from personal heartbreak and an unrelated but simultaneous career disappointment. Every day she spent two hours commuting on public buses to get to her new office, mostly because she didn't yet have enough money to buy herself a car. I didn't know it at the time, but Dr. Valero and I were both neck-deep in the messy business of creating new lives for ourselves. Maybe I sensed that on some level. Maybe that's partly why I trusted her so much. She didn't just know the science of my cancer and naturopathic care—she could see the real me.

I was one of Dr. Valero's first patients in her new practice, and already her most severe case. She recalls that I came to my first post-chemo appointments still struggling to stand and walk. My shins and calves hurt, and my hands and toes ached and peeled, as if they'd been badly sunburned—all side effects of the chemo. She remembers me telling her that my hands looked like they'd aged by a hundred years.

My cancer had been so advanced that my doctors had decided to pummel my system with chemo over a very short period of time. Thankfully, my immune system had held out just enough to withstand it and overcome tumor lysis syndrome.

Now I needed to rebuild my immunity from the ground up. The process hurt in a very literal sense, revealing aches and pains that rippled throughout my body almost nonstop.

Each time I arrived for a new treatment, Dr. Valero would mix a bag and set me in a chair, where I would watch Netflix while that day's IV dripped into me to perform its ninja magic. During one of my early treatments, I arrived with a bad cold and a moderate to severe case of panic. One specific blood marker that my doctors had been tracking closely had recently increased, and a nurse at the outpatient hospital cancer clinic had told me it could only be caused by cancer. Frightened by the news, I shared it with Dr. Valero, who promptly reassured me that the elevation in that particular marker could be easily attributed to my cold. It was a common reaction, even for someone without cancer. I could take a deep breath and focus on my recovery.

Seeing Life through a New Lens

As I navigated the ups and downs of my newly emerging life, everything slowly began to feel brighter. I was seeing the world in Technicolor hues I'd never let myself notice. There was hope and possibility now, and it was all around me. I could make decisions. I could be myself and do all the things I'd wanted to do but had never let myself try. There would be no more sitting on the fence thinking about what I wanted to do; it was time to do what I yearned to do. I would never feel fulfilled or even satisfied with a "regular" life. I was seeking more—I always had been—and now I would turn it all into real action, quantifiable steps.

Finally, I gave myself permission to do all the things I'd always wanted to do, but never allowed myself to. Paddle-boarding, taking spontaneous weekend trips, running, camping, cooking, sweating in infrared saunas—all of that and more called to me. This, it seemed, was what living was meant to be—a challenging, thrilling adventure that I either had to seize every day or give up altogether.

Out of the blue, I'd feel a yearning to go somewhere. Without warning, I'd announce to the kids on a random Friday afternoon that we were taking a trip. A few hours later, we'd be packed into our beat-up old van, ready for the open road. Sometimes we'd go camping; other times, I'd start driving without having a clue where we'd end up. It turned out it didn't matter if I'd made plans in advance or not. We'd sing, laugh, and have a blast, regardless. We were free to do whatever sounded like fun. This was what living was meant to feel like. How had I not realized that?

All of it cost money, of course, but again and again, in spite of the odds, I found the six hundred dollars to buy a used paddleboard, and the eight hundred I needed to get the puppy I'd always wanted. I named our Bernese mountain dog Ellie, and even at a very young age, she outweighed Felix by several pounds. Numerous times I got calls from the gym saying my membership fee hadn't gone through. Every time there was another financial obstacle or setback, I'd find a way to renew my membership or pay the overdue fee.

Following through and making these purchases was new to me. I'd never dared to invest in myself before. Each new purchase helped me to heal my relationship with myself and with money. I finally felt deserving, willing and able to buy experiences and things that I desired, and also able to manifest what I wanted.

Putting a Stop to Self-Sabotage

Nothing was perfect, but I was making my new life work. While I didn't often stop long enough to notice how much I was doing, I did notice that time was passing. *You're one day closer to ten months, Heather... one week closer to ten months... keep going... you can't stop now.*

I tried not to worry that I still wasn't entirely well; that months after chemo and months into vitamin C therapy, I was still vomiting and still struggling to heal my body, overcome near-constant joint and bone pain, fight colds, and regain energy. Living that reality without obsessing about what it meant, or didn't mean, wasn't easy.

Why is this happening? Is the cancer back? Questions like these ran through my mind constantly, a subliminal chatter that was always threatening to put me back into a depressive state. Every day the magnetic pull toward the numbing effects of sleep, inertia, and inaction were very real and very intense. Whenever I'd give into it, deciding that a particular moment wasn't the time to push, I'd take a nap and then descend into a shame spiral. *You're failing, Heather. If you want to live, you have to fight for it.*

I constantly had to check myself, to notice how, where, and when I was self-sabotaging. I couldn't yet function at regular speed, but I also couldn't slow down too often or for too long; defaulting to rest would make it much, much harder to get up next time. *Go live, Heather. Be brave, Heather. No one said this would be easy. Get up and do something.*

There was no break and no easy way forward. I could succumb to inactivity and suffer from self-pity and shame, or I could fight to live and alternate between feeling exhilarated and terrified, exhausted and frustrated.

Being brave enough to make tough choices also applied to how I was showing up as a mother. Logan was scheduled to go to his first sleepaway camp that summer. Months earlier, when we'd registered him, it had seemed like a good idea. However, when the time came for him to leave for four nights, I felt very differently. Would he be safe? What if something happened to him? Every fiber in my being wanted to cuddle with him and hold him close. He, too, was anxious about leaving, and he was my baby, my firstborn. How could I let him go?

It was completely outside of my comfort zone, but I had to let him leave. If we were going to live, I had to let my children do things that were healthy for them, even when those things didn't immediately feel that way for me. By allowing him to go, I was also walking my talk, showing him how to be brave in the face of fear. It was agonizing, but important too.

Up-Leveling

Being brave was also a dominant theme in growing my business. When I was asked to speak at a conference in New Jersey, I was too afraid to fly, so instead Bryan and I spent hours in the car.

Sitting in the passenger seat watching the world go by, I still didn't know what I was going to say. I also didn't have anything to wear onstage, so on the way we stopped at a mall. I bought some clothes, although not ones that I felt like myself in. My hair was still very short, my body was still healing in uncomfortable ways, and money was tight. Spending money and energy finding the "right" clothes didn't yet feel worthwhile.

The conference seemed like a good opportunity—to practice speaking and hopefully get a new client or two—but I wasn't at all sure if I would have anything interesting to say. Since finishing chemo, I'd continued coaching clients one-on-one, picking up a few more as I went along. I was also doing webinars and starting to work on launching my own podcast.

What had been an expensive hobby was turning into an actual business, but I still had a long way to go, and now, an hour onstage to say something memorable.

I decided to call my talk "Energetic Time Management." That name, and the practice it eventually became, is one that I now teach to help women manage their energy, not their time. That day, however, I did minimal preparation, got up onstage, and began talking. I told my story and eventually figured out the point I was making. Afterward, I tried to respond graciously when people came up to tell me how great my talk had been. *What was so great about it?* I kept thinking. *That was a disaster!*

AT THAT same event, I met the tough-as-nails woman who would become my next coach. I'm not scared easily, but honestly, this woman *terrified* me. She was all business, no warmth, and unbelievably intimidating. She also cost more than I could even dream of spending on a coach, but yet again, I found a way to make it work.

I won't pretend that we became best friends, but to this day she remains one of the most significant mentors I've ever had. Over and over again, she called me on my bullshit. "Heather, do you even want to make money?" she'd ask, clearly irritated by my anxiety and hesitation. Any and every excuse I made to avoid up-leveling my business and my work fell on deaf ears with her. She was having none of it. While her harsh demeanor eventually became too much for me, I'm endlessly grateful for the blunt and brutal honesty she served up. She showed me what it meant to get serious about my success.

My Other Office

After completing chemo, I arrived home one day to find an expensive water purification system waiting for me by my front door. There was a note attached. Neviana, the owner of the local café that had made me food while I was in the hospital, had done enough fundraising to purchase the system for us. Thanks to her, I would have pure water to drink, a crucial benefit for anyone who's as immune compromised as I was.

I'd been an occasional customer of the café prior to my diagnosis, and now, even more so. I liked it there. I could eat healthy food, and the atmosphere was always positive. As my energy ebbed and flowed, it became my office away from home. Two or three times a week, I'd go there with my laptop. Sometimes I'd ask Neviana if she could make me oatmeal, even when it wasn't on the menu, because it seemed like the only food I'd be able to stomach.

Neviana is a great cook and very knowledgeable about healthy food. We began to talk here and there, and she soon became a great resource. When I wanted to do a juice cleanse, I asked her which juicer I should buy. When I heard about a new healthy eating or recipe book, I'd ask her what she thought about it. It turned out, she'd signed up for my email list before I'd even been diagnosed, hoping to get support for an issue she was facing as a mom. As I began turning to her to learn more about health, food, and cooking, she began coming to me for emotional support.

We shared an easy rapport and a compatible sense of humor. She'd sometimes pass my table and make a fart noise just loud enough for me to hear. When she'd bring my oatmeal, I'd ask her if she was poisoning me, hoping to make me crap my pants that night. Eventually our in-the-café friendship extended outside its walls, and we began to go to hot yoga classes at night. I was super flexible and she wasn't, and we quickly learned not to look at each other during class to avoid cracking up for no particular reason.

As my dream of growing my business turned into reality, I turned to her for a new kind of support. I wanted to start hosting retreats for my growing list of clients and followers. Would she cater my events? Before long, Neviana's food came on boats, to hotels, and to cabins in the woods. Wherever I was hosting a retreat, Neviana would join me and elevate the event with her amazing food. It remains a staple of my events, even now as I write this.

Crossing the Finish Line

Finally, the day came. Statistically, I was out of the danger zone. Ten months had passed since I'd finished chemo. My body was healing. I could take a breath, feel some sense of relief.

During those months, Dr. Valero had kept a close eye on my blood work, my symptoms, and my mindset. When I had asked her if I could stop the vitamin C treatments prematurely, she'd firmly said no. By that point she knew me and my big plans to expand my career and ramp up my life in almost every way. Recognizing that my propensity to go, go, go was connected to my desire to live, she never asked me to scale back my plans. Instead, she dutifully maintained and sometimes increased my preventive care, readying my body for what my mind had planned next.

As I crossed the ten-month threshold, I wasn't just ready to fly. I was ready to soar, knowing full well that only some parts of my journey would feel smooth.

End of Chapter Exercise: The Art of Asking

One of the many important lessons that cancer taught me was the art of asking. For months after chemo, the logistics of daily life were more than I could handle. Week after week, I was forced to reach out to people and ask for what I needed.

Can you be on standby to pick up my children today if I'm not feeling well? Can you take one of my children to practice this week? Next time you're at the store, can you pick up some groceries for me?

I tried to spread my requests around to avoid overwhelming anyone; but even then, asking for the help I needed continued to feel uncomfortable. That discomfort is a common experience for women. So many of us struggle with asking for the help we need, even when we know we need it.

Ladies, it's time for us to stop this madness! We do so much and take care of so many. We *have to* start creating space for ourselves and each other to ask for and receive the help we need. It's not only essential to our health and well-being, it's also an important way for us all to come together and create communities of women who are connected and actively participating in each other's self-actualization and success. Really and truly, it takes a village, and when we come together as women, for women, we can do anything.

Learning to ask for help isn't difficult. What we tend to struggle with is what we tell ourselves that getting help means, as well as how we feel about ourselves when we ask for it. What do you say to yourself about yourself when you ask for help? Start by noticing your self-talk so that you can begin repairing your relationship with receiving.

Ultimately, for the experience to feel easier, we also have to learn to ask for help without expecting to get it exactly how, when, where, and from whom we imagine. We have to learn to ask for help while accepting that no one has a responsibility to give us the help we need, precisely when, how, and where we need it. In other words, we have to learn to ask without expectation, and with love, acceptance, and understanding when people can't meet our needs.

Like so much in life, asking for help, as well as digesting the idea that we won't always get the help we need how, when, and where we want it, takes practice. As with most practices, asking for help is about starting small. Begin by asking someone to start a load of laundry or open a door for you when your arms are filled with grocery bags. Over time, that can turn into asking someone to wash and fold laundry or bring the groceries inside and put them away. It can also mean training people to support you in your business, first in small ways, then in more significant ones.

Find one new thing you can get help with every day and then ask for it. You won't always get the help you need, but even then, you need to continue asking. Above all, start small and commit to asking for help daily with one new task or from one new person.

9

Looking Back, Living Forward

MY FIRST CANCER-FREE anniversary came and went, and throughout, my business continued to take off. It was exhilarating, but also overwhelming in ways I never imagined. I was doing interviews, growing my email list and social media following, and adding to my online community group and list of coaching clients too. It was all happening. My dream, and all the growth it required, was becoming real.

In January 2015, I sat down in my office with my new recording equipment all set up. It was time to record my first podcast. I was terrified. What would I say? Would I sound stupid? Would anyone even listen to it? I'd already put off recording my first episode for weeks, but finally I recorded it, posted it online, and left it, too full of angst and dread to create a second episode. Finally, a few weeks later, I checked and saw that eight people had downloaded it. *Eight people have listened to my interview.* That idea felt surreal at the time.

My podcast audience started small, but I was determined to make it grow. Sometimes I'd prepare for an episode in advance, but most often, I'd delay for weeks, feeling unsure what to say and insecure that whatever I did say would be interesting. Finally, after days of debating with myself while gnawing on uncomfortable emotions—*Should I prepare something or just show up and get it done? Ugh . . . I really don't want to do this . . .*—I'd remind myself that I'd made a commitment not to give up. After minimal preparation, or more often no preparation at all, I'd make myself sit down, hit record, and just . . . talk.

One episode at a time, it eventually added up to something—not that it felt that way for the first couple of years. Finally, though, a few years into it, my podcast reached over one million downloads. In 2020, we surpassed the four-million-downloads mark. It's still hard to believe that it all started that one day, me sitting in my office talking, scared out of my mind as I clicked the record button on my computer and began, "Alright, Mama, welcome . . . to the *Mom Is In Control* podcast."

Resisting the Pace of Healing

As I moved deeper into recovery, I grew increasingly irritated by the pace of my healing. I wanted, above all, to *live*, and living meant putting cancer firmly in my past. After regaining a lot of my strength and stamina, I decided to push myself further and try CrossFit, which is a high-intensity interval training regimen that a friend of mine had been raving about. Stepping up my fitness game felt like an important step forward, and I showed up consistently, not just literally and physically, but mentally too.

I *liked* being challenged. I *wanted* to be challenged. Challenging my mind and body with a new workout felt inspiring. It had very little to do what my body looked like. More than anything, I yearned to live beyond the limitations of my health. I wanted to feel free, to know that my body was mine again.

"Heather, your 20 percent is like most people's 100 percent," my trainer remarked one day as I once again pushed myself to get stronger and faster.

I looked at him, confused.

"You don't need to go this hard every time. It's okay to work out at a lower intensity sometimes."

I nodded, feeling defeated but also aware that he was saying something that I needed to hear. The truth was, CrossFit was more than my body could handle at that point. Fairly quickly after adhering to this workout regimen, my body had responded with painful ear infections and hard-to-get-rid-of colds. Once again, my body speaking to me. *Not this much, Heather, Slow down, Heather.*

Would I ever be able to live a full life, or would my health hold me back forever?

It was incredibly frustrating, but also important information. As much as I hated to admit it, my body wasn't back to normal yet. It had endured a boatload of chemo in a very short period of time. I'd felt a lot better after the first round of chemo, but the subsequent rounds had felt toxic, as if my body was being zapped of its life force.

Undeniably, I was one of the lucky ones. As advanced as my cancer had been, they'd been able to eliminate it with chemo. I was grateful—my cancer was gone—but my immune system needed more time to rebuild itself. The vitamin C infusions were doing a lot to protect me, but even after all this time had passed, my healing still wasn't happening at the pace I'd hoped it would.

I also hadn't gotten my period in months, which meant that my hormones were still out of balance. However, my scariest symptom was the occasional abdominal bloating I'd experience. Each time, I'd go into a tailspin of controlled panic. *Is the cancer back? Why am I bloated? What does the bloat mean?*

During my first year post-chemo, I'd continued to appreciate how important it was for me to eat whole foods. Quick options like chips and other processed foods had a very real impact on my digestive system. Increasingly, I was making a point of eating food that nourished me. At times it felt hard— like a "project" I had to take on—but I also was finally realizing just how crucial nutritious food was to my healing journey.

Digesting My Past

Each morning I'd open my eyes suddenly to find my heart racing and my breathing shallow. Within seconds I'd break out in a sweat, feeling entirely unable to calm my mind or my body.

It was 2015, and while my podcast grew and our home life returned to a more normal state, I found myself waking up, day after day, to crushing panic attacks. On a surface level, it made no sense; I should have felt relieved. After all, my boys still had a living, breathing mother and would for a long time to come. I also still had Dr. Valero working to strengthen my immune system and keep a watchful eye on my body and my health. That space to breathe, that opportunity to pause and be grateful, was a huge gift, but also, it gave my primitive brain a chance to open the floodgates to a massive amount of emotion I'd been unknowingly holding in.

Throughout my treatment and recovery to date, I'd been through emotional ups and downs, to be sure. I'd had my long dark nights, both in and out of the hospital. However, through most of it, I'd stayed as strong and steady as I could. For my children, Bryan, and my business, that had felt important. It had also reminded me how much I had to live for. Throughout it all, I'd focused on what I needed to *do*—get up to eat breakfast with the kids before school, show up for my clients, get regular vitamin C injections from Dr. Valero, exercise, and so on. That strategy had been helpful—I was now cancer-free and growing stronger—but what I hadn't yet faced, not really, were my emotions.

Now that I was cleared to live and my body was healing, all of the emotions I'd been avoiding since my diagnosis came tumbling out. My body had been through major trauma, but so had my heart and spirit. On a deep soul level I couldn't control, I went through a process of emotional release that lasted for months. It was an intense time, when I was forced to digest enormous waves of anxiety that overcame me just as suddenly as a tsunami, and with as little warning.

Owning My Shit

Why isn't Bryan making more money? Why isn't he being more of a go-getter at work?

With debt still piling up, money stress sometimes felt overwhelming, and I'd have thoughts like these. At first, they would seem like legitimate questions. More often than I care to admit, I'd voice them to Bryan. Eventually, however, I'd catch myself and look inward. *Stop deflecting, Heather. You're the one with the big dreams. You're the one who's always wanted to make more money. Stop playing safe. It's time for you to really go for it.*

Owning your own mental or emotional baggage, which I affectionately refer to as "your shit," is incredibly uncomfortable. Blaming other people for our problems is so much easier. Throughout 2015 and 2016, as my external life transformed in ways it never had before, my shit was coming up in all kinds of new ways.

As I processed my pent-up emotions post-recovery, I realized how important it was for me to practice what I was preaching to my clients and in my business—which meant I had to own my shit in more ways than I cared to. In addition to anxiety, I was still angry about feeling like I always had to be the one to stay strong for others. I also resented having had to play that role even when I'd had stage four cancer, even while undergoing chemo and throughout my recovery.

I could blame other people, sure. That's always an option; but it was also one that would take me away from the bigger vision I'd committed to. What was becoming clearer to me was that I was still learning how to truly feel my emotions. That would require me to be vulnerable, and vulnerable was not something I wanted to be. That resistance, I knew, was a teacher unto itself, showing me which path to choose in order to be the woman I'd always known I could be and live the life I'd always dreamed of living.

Evolving toward Worthiness

Some people see chemo as poison. I'd never fully trusted Western medicine, so I'd had serious reservations as well. Cancer is big business, without question, and chemo is a part of that. However, when I was diagnosed, I didn't have time to research alternate options. I was dying, and quickly. In spite of some friends' recommendations that I pursue only natural cancer treatments, I decided to proceed with chemo. However imperfect, chemo proved to be essential to my survival, and I was grateful for each treatment I got. In fact, each time I had one, I looked at the chemo bag and silently said, "Thank you. I'm open to receiving your healing."

When I look back on it now, I see those hours I spent receiving chemo's healing as the start of a longer and more profound journey. Up until that point, I'd neglected my most basic need for nourishment—food, as well as other kinds—for so long that chemo was my only option. Even before our community had hosted those two fundraisers on our behalf, chemotherapy had begun teaching me how to receive.

Now in my post-recovery years, I was finally feeling stronger and consciously up-leveling my life in all kinds of ways. At long last it was time to face the core issue behind my resistance to receiving—my deep feelings of shame and unworthiness.

At a young age I'd internalized a core belief that I was unworthy and always would be. It hurt so badly that by my teen years, I'd wanted to die. Throughout my childhood, I hadn't had strong female role models I could relate to, or who I felt could nurture and guide me. Being a rebel, I'd also attracted a lot of criticism from teachers and other authority figures. Although I'd probably projected a strong exterior, deep down it had all hurt.

Given this, it may seem ironic that I later set out to become a social worker advocating for children in need. Really, however, it had been a subconscious way of trying to help others while also healing my own deep emotional wounds. It's so easy for children to look like they're "fine" and slip through the cracks. I would know; in many ways I'd been one of those children. On some level I'd hoped that "saving" other children might also make my pain go away.

It hadn't worked, of course. I'd been unable to "save" those children or escape my own private pain. That's not how life works.

Becoming pregnant with Logan had forced me to stop waiting for someone to nurture me and show me the way forward. Knowing I would become a mother had forced me to figure out how to get my act together on my own. It had been challenging but becoming a mother had also given me a reason to live. For years afterward, Logan, and then Calvin and Felix, too, had been my Big Why. He, and then they, had inspired me to get up each day, to get through school, to grow my business, and to do whatever was necessary to create a good life so they didn't have to suffer as I had.

What I eventually had to learn the hard way is that living for other people ultimately doesn't work; that eventually we each have to face the one person we've always known and will always live with—ourselves. I'd resisted that basic and obvious truth so deeply and for so long that I'd almost died when my youngest was barely beginning to walk. Now that I was getting a second chance at life, I was learning how to live, but in order to succeed at it, I was also having to face the fact that I still didn't feel worthy. No matter how my life looked from the outside, I still didn't *feel* like I was enough.

The Darkness in the Limelight

Western society has a distorted view of success. We talk about "stepping into the limelight" as if it's some magical gift. It comes with its pluses, for sure, but most everyone I know who has felt this "light" has logged a lot of hours getting there. That was true of me too. As I put in my own sweat and tears, however, I was realizing that the work wasn't the hard part. The true challenge of becoming more visible, of realizing my dreams and succeeding at higher levels, was feeling I deserved any of the applause, attention, or success.

As my client base and social media following grew, more people began to express their desire to be like me and to achieve a similar level of success. I was grateful for all of it, but also struggling with my new reality. Higher levels of success and visibility also translate into more activity and abundance, but with that comes more work and more attention, only some of which is positive.

The more I challenged myself, the more I was surrounded by people even more successful than I was. The more followers

I got, the more feedback I received. When I achieved a big business goal, I'd find myself surrounded by industry leaders who'd achieved a lot more than I had, and in less time. When I spoke on social media about a struggle I was having with my body, I'd get comments about the "new" mindfulness or eating regimen I "should" be doing. No matter what I did or how much of myself I gave, none of it ever felt "good" enough.

None of this was happening for negative reasons or specifically to hurt me, but when you harbor deep feelings of shame, even well-intended critiques—or what I call love taps—sometimes hurt. That applied to my podcast too, even as my following grew by leaps and bounds. Unable to control my potty mouth, I'd sometimes drop f-bombs and get very mixed reactions. Like clockwork, some mothers would email comments like, "I love your message, but you would make a bigger impact if you stopped swearing. This is inappropriate for a parenting podcast," while at the same time I'd be getting emails from other mothers who'd say that my f-bombs were when they knew I was "their girl."

What became so clear as I grew my business and got more feedback was that I only wanted success if I could achieve it on my terms. That meant sounding like a truck driver sometimes—even if some people felt it was inappropriate. (My "explicit" episodes have grown fewer and farther between over time, but sometimes dropping f-bombs is just what our souls need.) It also meant being my unscripted self and being more vulnerable online and on my podcast, in spite of the fact that sharing more of myself was leaving me more open to judgment.

Criticism stung at times, yes, but little by little, I realized that I could get over these hurt feelings. I could recover from those little love taps and still stay true to the only person I'd ever wanted to be: me. The question I began to face was, how did I feel about her?

The Silent Killer

Unfortunately, shame is all too easy to implant in the tender hearts and minds of children. Abuse, abandonment, and trauma are obvious sources of shame. The more common sources, many of which are often overlooked, include cultural biases, such as racism, as well as negative commentary, name-calling, and labeling—as the "smart one" or the "troublemaker," et cetera—that place children in boxes not of their own making. Over time, these subtler forms of shaming can completely take away a child's hope.

While I never suffered from the shame imposed upon children by racism, I was one of countless children whose deep feelings of shame and unworthiness slipped under the radar. It's a danger that we, as girls and women, are especially susceptible to. From a young age, we're taught that nourishing ourselves—not just with food, but with self-love, self-actualization, creativity, attention, self-compassion—is taking away from others. In obvious as well as more subtle ways, we internalize the idea that self-sacrificing makes us more worthy. When we become mothers, we tell ourselves that always caring for our children first is what we're supposed to do, what we have to do; that caring for our children first and foremost is what will make each of us a "good" mother. As time passes, these beliefs become more ingrained, and even as our children grow older and more capable, self-sacrifice remains our default.

Why, ladies, why? Why are we so dedicated to this way of living when we know it makes us feel unloved, resentful, impatient, anxious, and under-realized? Why are we so committed to measuring our worth according to how much of our selves we sacrifice?

Once I had a better handle on who I was and wanted to be, these questions swirled around inside me, poking and prodding at my deeper emotions and beliefs, my ingrained habits and assumptions. More and more, I found my life and my experiences shaping my message. If I was going to be the kind of woman, mom, and coach I'd always wanted to be, I had to share struggles on my podcast and my social media, even when that meant receiving judgment and criticism in return.

Seeking Nourishment

Women were resonating with what I was saying, but as grateful as I was for my growing success, it didn't always feel how I wanted it to feel. Why was that? Why couldn't I enjoy my success and my life more?

As I barreled forward, determined to challenge myself and grow toward my discomfort rather than shrink from it, I ran again and again into the core lesson my cancer had taught me: When I self-sacrifice—when I value what I give to others above and beyond my own needs and desires—I leak energy. Creatively, emotionally, intellectually, energetically, spiritually, and physically, I end up in a state of chronic malnourishment. I empty myself out and in the process deplete all that I would otherwise have to offer others.

Value yourself, Heather. Stop selling yourself short.

As I continued to take a stand for myself and my bigger hopes and dreams—for my children and my career and also my health, happiness, and ability to feel safe and at ease in my own skin—I had to repeat things like this to myself often. I still wasn't practicing enough self-nourishment; the more I achieved, the more self-nourishment I required. That was obvious on an intellectual level, but emotionally, it was incredibly challenging prioritizing my needs and desires above others'. I, like so many of my clients and followers, had always measured my self-worth according to how much I was self-sacrificing. Now, finally, I could see so clearly how much that desire to please and "save" others was tamping down my own joy and well-being, and in turn limiting how much I had to give.

At long last, the message I'd most needed to hear came through clearly—to be a "good" mother to my children and our world, as well as a good steward of my hopes and dreams, I first had to nurture myself. I had to nourish Heather physically, emotionally, and spiritually so I could show up for my family and the life I wanted to live.

Accepting What Is

I'd love to be able to tell you that self-nourishing is all about pleasure and enjoyment, like getting pedicures and taking long, soulful walks with close friends. While those activities and more sometimes factor into self-nourishment, the real work is something else altogether. We'll dive more deeply into that work in Part III of this book, but what I found during my post-recovery years was that a lot of it was about acceptance.

When we commit to ourselves, which also means committing to self-nourishing and self-actualizing, we simultaneously have to face our truth. When we go for our dreams, we're forced to face the previous dreams that didn't pan out, the relationship we thought we'd have, the children we imagined raising, and the life we envisioned ourselves living. It's a lot, especially when we're simultaneously expanding our lives, as I was. When we harbor shame, we also tend to turn our disappointments and heartbreaks back on ourselves, telling ourselves we're the problem; we're not worthy enough or lovable enough, and so on.

Byron Katie has famously said, "It's not your job to like me— it's mine." That challenge—to truly like myself—soon became my most powerful growing edge. Katie's work, aka The Work, was an invaluable tool during these years, helping me to process and release the emotional residue I'd let pile up inside me for so many years. Whenever I noticed myself descending into a shame spiral, I'd pull out one of her worksheets and fill it out. They helped me enormously, giving me a chance to become aware of how I was feeling, the stories I was telling myself, and the new beliefs I could choose instead.

The Work is never done, of course, and what I learned most of all during this time was the power of acceptance. The more I was able to accept myself and my life as it was— disappointments, home runs, missteps, and all—the more I was able to show up for myself and then my loved ones, my clients, and my life.

PART III

Living to Be a Good Mother

10

Your "Problem" Child Is Your Greatest Gift

AS I CONTINUE to expand my coaching business, helping greater numbers of women through my podcast, online courses, and in-person events, I see the common threads in our individual stories so clearly. Some of those common threads are experiences we tuck away, hoping no one will notice them. One of those is yelling at our kids, and then sinking, yet again, into shame, fear, guilt, and worry. Desperate to regain some sense of control in their homes and with their children, women come to me seeking a new way forward. Almost without exception, these mothers have a "problem" child, the one who consistently pushes their most vulnerable, combustible buttons, the one who escalates the already considerable challenges of motherhood, piercing like an arrow aimed at their squishiest, mushiest spots.

What most of my clients are surprised to discover is that their "problem" child is also a guiding light pointing them toward the journey they most need to undertake. That journey is the one I began when Logan was born, and also the one we'll begin in this chapter and continue through the end of this book. It's ultimately about learning to trust and value yourself, which is how you'll find the inner knowing and clarity to transform your entire experience around parenting, as well as your relationship with yourself and your children.

The Paradox of Motherhood

As mothers, we're unavoidably judged, both as parents and through other people's views of our children. The offhand comments, the looks, and the "helpful suggestions" may come from friends, family, schools, and neighbors. When we have a child who's different in some way, the pain of these judgments can feel especially acute. Too often, they taint how we see our children as well as how we see ourselves as mothers.

When we get caught in this cycle of judgment, it's partly because we've consciously or unconsciously bought into the idea that there's a "right" way to parent. In that mindset, we may then forget to notice how many different and conflicting beliefs there are around what it even means to be a "good" mother. Here's a list of just some of the beliefs about motherhood—often in contradiction—that I've encountered over the years, both as a mother and coach:

- Our children should be perfect, because, naturally, our parenting is, too, or it should at least look or sound or seem that way.

- Parenting causes perpetual exhaustion, dirty hair days, bad hair days, body confidence issues, and endless feelings of overwhelm. It also creates the need for nonstop caffeine and, of course, "wine o'clock."

- Parenting is hard, and if you don't complain about it or feel miserable, exhausted, and stressed out most of the time, you're not one of the "good" moms.

- Yelling at your children is shameful and admitting to it is even more so.

- Everyone yells at their children, and if you don't, you're not a "real" mom. It's the only way to get these pesky, entitled children to listen.

- Even raising your voice with your child is a form of abuse and something you should never do.

- If you have a "problem" child, or if your child is different in any way, it's embarrassing and also your fault, as their parent.

- Even feeling like you have a "problem" child reflects poorly on you as a mother. You should love your children and be proud of them, not blame them.

- Everyone has a "problem" child—get in line and join the club! That's parenting for you—you give your all and never get a break.

Ladies, we can't win if we're trying to become someone else's idea of a "good" mother! The moment we satisfy one definition of "good," we go against another. It's a lose-lose proposition.

Also, our children are unique souls. They deserve to be parented according to their own needs. Who could possibly assess your child's needs better than you?

On a deeper level, we already know all of this, of course, but still we overextend ourselves trying to be the kind of "good" mother we think we're supposed to be. Why do we do this? Why do we torture ourselves trying to meet expectations and standards that aren't even our own?

"I Do Know"

One of the reasons we buy into this idea that everyone else's opinion of our children and our parenting matters so much is the lie so many of us tell ourselves. That lie is this: "I don't know."

When we default to "I don't know," we invalidate our inner knowing and make other people's opinions and ideas more important than our own. When this becomes a pattern in our parenting, we may allow ourselves to be overly influenced by people who don't know or understand us or our children as well as we do.

To be clear, when I say that "I don't know" is a lie, I'm *not* suggesting that we need to know everything, or that we already know how to handle every situation we encounter as a parent or in any other part of our lives. If you've read the chapters before this one, you already know how much I believe in learning to ask for what we need. However, too often when we're faced with a challenge or problem, we default to "I don't know" to avoid what's really happening inside us.

In spite of all my years of personal development work and coaching, I recently fell into this trap. As I co-create these chapters, the COVID-19 pandemic is beginning to overtake our lives. Tens of millions of people are out of work, our children are virtual- or homeschooling, and life as we've long known it is shape-shifting before our eyes in ways that don't feel clear or comforting. While my business and family are well-prepared financially (check out my podcast for more on how we did that), my short-term vision and goals feel anything but secure. I'm grateful for many things, and so far I've stayed focused on living, loving, working, and helping those in need as much as I can, but still, the uncertainty sometimes feels overwhelming. Like most, I've cycled through a wide range of emotions. It's been interesting to observe.

Even with our world so up in the air, I knew that the problem was inside me; that I couldn't blame "things that are happening" or the kids being home all the time. This obstacle I was facing was inside me. Knowing that, I focused on adjusting my business plans for the remainder of 2020, but still reached a point of feeling lost. What programs did I still want to offer? How should I change them? When should I launch each one? There were so many questions, and in the midst of all the confusion, I kept running into that same mental wall: *I don't know.*

Then one morning, I had a breakthrough. It started with an online morning yoga class I'd promised myself I'd take. Honestly, though, when 7 a.m. came, I had zero interest. At that moment, I would have considered vomiting all day over doing this class—really any excuse would have been fine with me.

You need this, Heather. Just show up.

I pushed myself to go and for at least the first fifteen minutes of class, I was completely in my head, resisting every pose and every breath. My exercise bra also didn't fit right, and I'd somehow managed to wear my ugliest, least favorite T-shirt. Feeling heavy and unattractive, I soon realized that I was flashing my boobs every time I did a new pose. Embarrassed, I put on a sweatshirt, only to get so hot I felt like I was suffocating. Torn between heat-induced suffocation and the humiliation of exposing my boobs to a group of strangers online, I put my sweatshirt on, then took it off. This happened multiple times within a ten-minute period. Finally, the yoga teacher called me out and asked what was going on. I explained, apologized, and then decided enough was enough. It was time to focus on yoga.

A few minutes later, I was doing poses and thinking a lot less about where my boobs were. After class, everything felt a little bit better, as if a cloud of dark emotions had been lifted off me. Grateful that I'd pushed myself to show up in spite of my resistance, I showered and put on just enough makeup to perk myself up before starting my first Zoom meeting of the day. As I began talking, I realized that my "I don't know" was a mask for the emotional turmoil I'd been feeling. In fact, I knew very well what I needed to do, both for myself and my business. I'd just temporarily fallen into the "I don't know" trap to avoid feeling my emotions. Once I'd gotten back into my body and out of my head, I could easily move back into a place of flow.

What "I Don't Know" Actually Means

As women, we often "I don't know" ourselves around our own parenting. So many clients have confessed to feeling confident at work and throughout much of their lives—except for when it comes to parenting. As soon as they walk into their own homes and face their children, they tell me that their sense of self seems to vanish.

As mothers, we default to self-doubt after a challenging or upsetting interaction with our children and then assume it's because we don't know how to parent our children. In reality, though, we know a lot more about our children and our parenting than we realize. When we say "I don't know," what we're actually doing is avoiding feeling complicated emotions like fear, shame, and anxiety.

What "I don't know" really means is that we first need to check in with ourselves and figure out how we're feeling. Why is it important to take this time to ourselves first, before seeking input from family and friends? When we're feeling overwhelmed, that is sometimes reflected back to us. By placing more value on asking others for their ideas, we're valuing their input over our own; basically, we're prioritizing their ideas and feelings above our own emotions and desires. When we do this, we give our power away and sometimes also set ourselves up to be judged in ways that don't serve us.

When we acknowledge "I don't know" as an invitation to pause and get clearer on how we're feeling and what we actually do (and don't) know, we can then seek input from others from a more centered and focused place.

We'll look at how to do this in the coming chapters, but first let's talk about how this relates to having a "problem" child.

The "Problem" Child

Isobel is one of my clients who comes to mind as a woman who felt she didn't know how to handle her "problem" child. A successful corporate executive and married mother of four children, she came to me with a severe case of burnout. In addition to being the primary breadwinner in her household, she had a demanding job in a male-dominated corporate culture. For years she'd been feeling weighed down by the pressure to "do it all."

Too overwhelmed to continue living as she had been, Isobel had begun a sabbatical year from her job just before we met. She sought me out to learn new ways to manage her youngest daughter's extreme sensitivity to the outside world and to set healthy emotional boundaries for her oldest daughter, who was preparing to leave for college.

Still elementary school–aged, her youngest had been diagnosed with autism. Feeling pressured to show up as a parent how others seemed to expect her to, Isobel found herself yelling at her youngest and then spiraling down into shame and self-doubt. With her oldest daughter, she felt afraid of letting go and losing her. Even without her job on her mind, these parenting challenges felt like a lot to handle.

Especially with her youngest daughter, the pressure Isobel was feeling from others was overshadowing her own maternal instincts and making her feel like she "didn't know" how to parent that daughter. The outside world's expectations were also convincing her that she "should" be teaching her daughter to act and react in certain ways.

While trying to reassess her parenting, she was also feeling called to find out who she was and what she wanted. For years she'd been living this big, successful-seeming life but feeling like she had little to no control over what happened in it. Eventually, she admitted to feeling so overwhelmed that she'd occasionally fantasize about veering off the road just to catch a break from her own life.

As we continued working together, she began to tap into her own instincts and create a completely different relationship with her youngest daughter. Just by tuning out the external world's judgments and getting more centered within herself, she was better able to tune into her daughter's needs. Instead of parenting from a reactionary place, she was able to understand her youngest's extreme sensitivities, even though the outside world typically couldn't. At the same time, Isobel began to parent her eldest daughter in new ways, giving her more space and independence while continuing to provide love and support.

Over time, Isobel also realized that she didn't have to be a "perfect" parent. That created space in herself and her life. Instead of fantasizing about veering off the road, she began to acknowledge her latent desire to support women in leadership positions.

Finally, after years of burning the candle at both ends, Isobel also began allowing herself to rest when she needed it.

Taking better care of herself ultimately gave her more energy and more capacity, both for herself and her family.

Beginning Your Journey

As a coach, my job is to help guide women to rediscover their inner knowing, but never to tell them what to do, how to parent, or how to live their lives. I couldn't possibly know that! I'm not you; your children aren't my children, and your life isn't my life.

When I first meet with women, almost all of whom are mothers, I ask them to describe what's happening, especially around their "problem" child. If they don't identify with that term, I simply ask them to remember a recent event when they felt triggered as a mother. Essentially, I need to get clear on why they're coming to me.

As you begin your own journey, that's also what you need to understand—why you're here, reading this book.

Take a moment now to jot down how your "problem" child triggers you or describe a recent exchange or event when you felt triggered as a mother. After describing what happened in as much detail as you can, ask yourself how you felt when you were triggered. Were you angry? Did you feel defeated? Frustrated? What was the primary emotion you felt once you were triggered? Don't worry about perfect. Just write down whatever comes to mind in your journal.

Redefining the "Problem" Child

Like Isobel, Jane came to me in a state of emotional overwhelm, feeling unable to manage her adopted son. As her "problem" child, he could push her buttons like no one else.

More often than she cared to admit, she resorted to yelling and scolding, only to feel ashamed afterward. It felt like they were on a downward spiral.

Jane had first met her son years earlier at an orphanage halfway around the world, and she'd immediately felt an intense, soul-level connection she couldn't ignore. At the end of her second visit, she brought him home. As he grew older, he began exhibiting different, often embarrassing, behaviors. Wherever they went, he seemed to attract negative attention, even scrutiny, from caregivers and other parents. This led to him being singled out at daycare and left out of kids' social events.

Jane felt perpetually conflicted, torn between wanting to stand up for her son, including his differences, and empathizing with others' impatience and irritation with her son's behavior. As the years piled up, she also began to feel frustrated and increasingly overwhelmed by her inability to teach him to conform to societal norms.

As we worked together, Jane, like Isobel, began to see that her son was showing her what she needed to see about herself. For years she'd been valuing others' opinions over and above her own. He was different, yes, but he'd also endured a lot of trauma since infancy. When she was able to cast aside others' views and expectations, she could once again feel the deep connection she and her son had always shared.

At the same time, she couldn't deny how much her sometimes frenetic energy was impacting her son's actions and reactions. By showing up and doing her own inner discovery work to calm and center herself, she realized that she could find new, more positive ways of being that could change how she was interacting with her son.

Resisting the Inner Discovery Process

Women often come to me wanting to talk at length about their "problem" child. When I redirect them toward themselves, many are initially resistant. They want solutions and quick-fix strategies around helping their child calm down or act and react differently.

I get it—motherhood can be overwhelming, and too many of us are running on mental, emotional, physical, and spiritual fumes. However, this is *your* life, and only you know and understand your child or children. This is not a plug-and-play child's behavior–control class. It's a self-discovery process that can, and will, transform your relationship with yourself and your children, if you show up and do the work, as I was forced to begin doing when I had Logan. Fast-forward to the present, and he's growing into a young man whose self-awareness comes through in his honest communication. I'm proud of who he is and who he's becoming every day. It all began with my willingness to show up and do the work on myself, first and foremost.

To be clear, doing the inner discovery work does *not* imply that you're in any way to blame for your child's choices, or that you can or should try to control your children. It's about how we show up as mothers and the impact it has on our relationships with our children.

I saw this play out repeatedly when I worked with children in social services. Almost without exception, the children would respond with defiance, anger, and ignoring behaviors when a social worker approached them with anxiety and fear or judgment, blaming and shaming. However, when an adult like me showed up and tried instead to create connection with those same children, their attitude would begin to shift. If I continued to give them space to feel seen and heard, we'd begin to create trust and mutual understanding, not because I was demanding them to do or say certain things, but because I was creating an environment where they could feel valued.

This same give-and-take of emotional energies happens in every parent-child relationship. As mothers, we put out energy and our kids respond. Our children also put out energy and then we respond to them. It's a constant flow that can be hard to manage when we feel disconnected from our inner wisdom.

Imagine that you could feel more emotionally centered on a regular basis. Are you open to the possibility that by changing your emotional state, you could find ways to transform how parenting feels? Are you willing to do the work to create more connected, loving relationships with yourself and your children?

This process is never about pushing yourself toward burnout. Nor does it ask you to always take on more or do more. Parenting is not about exhaustion, depletion, or conflict. Trust me when I say that so much positive transformation is possible! I am living, breathing proof of that.

With that said, if you still secretly just want a quick fix for your "problem" child, that's okay. I hope you'll keep reading anyway, and also listen to my podcast, *Mom Is In Control*, for additional perspectives.

Noticing Your Zones

Remember the red, yellow, and green zones we discussed in Chapter 4? They're just as relevant for children as they are for adults. Over the years, especially as my children have grown older, the zones have become a useful way to communicate our state of mind at any given moment, especially when we're venturing toward a yellow or red zone. In addition to creating self-awareness, using zones helps each of us to explain what we need and when we're feeling triggered and why.

Since I've developed a habit of noticing how I'm feeling physically, mentally, and emotionally, it's grown easier over the years to be honest with myself and others about which zone I'm actually in. If I'm hungry, tired, or stressed out, a simple everyday conversation or exchange can more easily push me into the yellow zone. Bigger underlying issues like burnout, loneliness, and anxiety also tend to push us toward our yellow and red zones faster.

While the zones can manifest differently from person to person, this chart describes some of the emotions associated with each zone:

Green zone	Yellow zone	Red zone
Calm, peaceful	Irritated	Angry
Focused	Irritable	Out of patience
Happy, upbeat	Growing impatient or out of patience	Hopeless
Patient	Frustrated	Sad
Joyful	Anxious	Very anxious
Open-minded	Grumpy	Harsh, critical
Content	Tired and/or hungry	Depleted

Take a moment to notice how you're feeling right now. Which zone are you in? Notice how your body feels and how you relate to your children when you're in this particular zone.

Recently I was reminded of how important it is to notice our zones. I was scrolling through Facebook one day when a friend's post caught my eye. She had posted about "mom rage," which had been highlighted in a *New York Times* article about moms feeling like they would physically explode from rage after months of quarantine. In response, she had commented that she could relate to the article, since she had "no patience left." This is a great example of a yellow zone experience. Feeling impatient is a clear indication that you're in your yellow zone. You can stay in this state for a prolonged period, inching little by little toward your red zone until, finally, you lose your cool and begin screaming at your children. That can then leave you feeling guilty and overwhelmed—as in, back in your yellow zone and heading toward another red zone outburst. However, if you can step back and see your growing impatience as a yellow zone indicator, you can make conscious choices that move you toward your green zone instead. For me sometimes that's walking away from a heated situation, drinking a glass of water, or reassessing whether I've scheduled enough downtime in my calendar.

Exploring Your Green, Yellow, and Red Zones

What do you experience in each of your zones? So many clients tell me they go from green to red "just like that," but we all go through the yellow zone on the way to red. By noticing what each zone looks like, you can begin to identify what the yellow zone looks and feels like for you and practice taking time for yourself when you find yourself there.

Personally, when I'm tired or haven't been consistent with healthy habits, I'm more prone to going from yellow to red much faster. In my yellow zone, I feel off—sluggish, mentally foggy, unmotivated, and overwhelmed.

Here are some journal prompts to help you notice how the zones play out:

- What does your red zone look and feel like, both in your life and in your body, mind, and emotions?
- What happens when you try to solve problems while in your red zone?
- What happens in your mind, body, and emotions right before you enter your red zone?
- How does your body feel right before you're in the red zone?
- What triggers most often take you out of your green zone?

Identifying and Managing the Zones

As you move forward in this process, whenever possible, make a note in your journal about which zone you're in, what may have triggered you, and how it feels. Over time this simple practice will remind you to stop and notice how you're feeling before you act, react, or interact.

As you get into the habit of noticing your zones, you can begin to understand how to manage them.

The *green zone* is the easiest zone to be in. This is where we're grounded, centered, and in a good mood. One goal with this journey is to get to a point where you're naturally spending more time in the green zone. Interestingly, once that happens, you probably won't notice. It just becomes your baseline, a "new normal."

The *yellow zone* can be both the hardest and most important zone to identify and notice. Most of us have learned how to seem fine outwardly when we're in the yellow zone. Truthfully, though, in the yellow zone we're a lot like a glowing ember. We haven't yet sparked a fire, but we're combustible. We may look or seem like we're cooling down when in fact we're getting hotter. It can be a confusing state to be in.

If we're in the yellow zone because we're cooling down after being the red zone, that's a sign that we still need more time to get centered. If we're in the yellow zone heading toward the red zone, we need to be even more aware of our energy and mood. That's often a good time to exercise, journal, or find some other way to process and release our emotions in ways that don't negatively impact our loved ones.

The *red zone* is the emotional "danger zone," so to speak. Unlike the yellow zone, where we may pretend that we're fine, in the red zone we're usually very aware of how aggravated, angry, or impatient we're feeling. It's also where we're most likely to lash out at our children and generally say and do things that we later regret. Most of us can go from the yellow to red zone very quickly, which is another reason that it's especially important to begin noticing how we feel when we're in the yellow zone.

By noticing which zone you're in at various times, you can begin to create more emotional self-awareness, which is one of the key foundations of this journey. Personally, I tend to go from my green zone into my yellow zone when I skip my morning routine for a few days in a row. When that happens, I often feel less energized and motivated. I also begin to feel the weight of stagnant emotions and less able to get ahead of my day, which causes anxiety and contributes to feelings of overwhelm. Those are all signals that something has slipped and it's time for me to get back on track.

In the next chapter, we'll look some of the beliefs that can get in the way of this self-discovery process, but first let's also begin observing when your "problem" child is in the different zones.

End of Chapter Exercise: Noticing Your Child's Zones

As you practice noticing when you're in the red, yellow, and green zones, it's also important to take note of how your zones and your child's zones look, sound, and feel. If you have several children, focus first on the child who triggers you most often. Later you can begin applying it to your other children too.

The best place to start is with the yellow zone, since it's the hardest to identify and where we need to be most aware of how we're feeling. Use these journaling prompts as often as you need to understand your yellow zone and your child's.

Understanding your yellow zone:

1. What happens in your body, and with your behavior and emotions, right before you start yelling?

2. What simple, accessible habit makes you feel grounded and alive? E.g., taking a walk, journaling, meditating, gardening, et cetera. (*Hint: Since we're conditioned to deprive ourselves of joy, this is probably an activity you tend to resist even though you often feel better after doing it.*)

Observing your child's yellow zone:

1. What do you notice about your child's behavior right before they have a meltdown?

2. What activity does your child naturally gravitate toward that makes them feel calmer? (E.g., Legos, being outside, playing with a pet, et cetera.)

11

Excuses, Excuses,
No More Excuses

"**I HAVE YOUNG CHILDREN.**"

"My partner won't let me spend the money."

"I don't have enough energy."

"I'm already so busy."

"My family needs me."

"I can't fit anything else in around my job."

For years I, too, invested myself 100 percent in my excuses. I was a mother, a student, a working parent. I had bills to pay, and always, *other* people to take care of. Like so many mothers, I fed myself last. I took care of myself last. I noticed how I was feeling last, if ever. Always, I was sure that I had to come last; that my value as a mother depended on my being in last place—or more often, no place at all—on my priority list.

What is it going to take for us to put ourselves on our own to-do lists? Will you do what I did and wait until you get a potentially fatal diagnosis? Are you willing to risk that much just to hold on to your excuses? Isobel, and many other clients like her, spent months, even years, fantasizing about getting into a car wreck just to catch a break. Is that what you're wait-ing for—sirens and an ER visit with potentially irreversible consequences?

Ladies, seriously—what will it take for us to stop investing more in our excuses than we do in ourselves? And what's that all about anyway?

The Ultimate Failure

Some women come to me after a health scare. Others claim to be seeking fulfillment or say they're itching to start a business. When I ask what's really going on, a familiar story often spills out.

The actual truth is, they're yelling at their children. Again. Still. Things can't go on the way they have been. Deep down they can't justify their continually raised voices, their perpet-ual impatience, and their growing inability to enjoy the smaller humans they ushered into this world. Their failure to be a "good" mother feels shameful and inexcusable, a taboo subject to be kept secret.

People refer to parenthood as the "hardest job in the world," but we also seem to share a belief that we don't say: that being a so-called bad mother is to be a bad human. For us, as women and nurturers, it is the ultimate sin, the one unforgivable, inex-cusable stain on us and our basic nature. For this reason, too many of us have spent years swallowing our shame and regret, hoping that next time, we won't yell; that next time, the unend-ing patience we're supposed to be blessed with will finally come to life inside us.

But how will this happen? When will this happen? We seem to want to will this transformation to life, but without actually admitting that we're facing this problem in the first place.

When Mindy first came to me, she, too, was struggling to admit just how overwhelmed she was feeling. With an infant and toddler at home, as well as a full-time career, her chronic inflammatory disease had flared up. She had recently returned from an extended visit abroad—a trip she had taken to seek much-needed healing. Her body was clearly speaking to her, begging her to find a new way to live her life. Yet after inquiring about coaching options, she explained her decision not to move forward this way: "I can't spend the money."

The money excuse is a complex issue in many ways. There are absolutely times when certain kinds of investments aren't in a person's best financial interest. There are also times when people, especially entrepreneurs, can make the money that they need to get the support they want. I've done that repeatedly over the years, including during cancer treatment and recovery, ramping up my marketing and increasing enrollments so I could afford what I needed to reach my goals. That ability to manifest more money within a relatively short amount of time is also a privilege; however, in this particular woman's case, it was clear that money wasn't the true obstacle she was facing. Instead, money was an easy excuse for Mindy to avoid the fact that she didn't feel sufficiently deserving of the support she needed. I took her response as an indication that she wasn't yet ready to be coached and wished her well.

A couple of years later, Mindy contacted me again, still looking for coaching. After years of communicating with her children through yelling and ultimatums, she'd had enough. She couldn't hear herself yell at her little ones anymore. She didn't want to continue threatening them with reduced privileges—less screen time, for example—in order to get them to comply with her. Finally tired of her own excuses, she was ready to get help and find a new way to live and parent.

Like Mindy, many of us know that we need to do something to stop ourselves from losing it the next time our children are defiant, distracted, or running late once again, yet we resist opportunities to seek the help we need. So often we do this

172 DYING TO BE A GOOD MOTHER

because we can't admit to ourselves, and certainly not to others, that we're yelling at our children in the first place. It's a secret we think of as too dark to share. However, after years of avoidance and denial, years of telling themselves that things will get better with time or other external changes, they finally come to me, confessing, but again only partially, that they may be part of the problem.

But what does that even mean—that we, as mothers, are "part of the problem"?

Defining the "Problem"

First things first—we are *not* fundamentally flawed. We are *not* bad humans for yelling at our children. We may need to look within, feel our feelings, take on new beliefs, and adjust our actions and behavior, but we are *not* broken, damaged, or deserving of blame.

The "bad" mother shame so many of us carry around is far more common than we realize. It's a trap that we can learn to avoid in the future, but it is not a stain on us, our character, or our worthiness as women, mothers, or humans. We do *a lot* of amazing things. What we don't do very well is recognize that fact and value ourselves.

When we look at why so many of us suffer in such similar ways, we find the real problem we've been facing all along—a need to self-sacrifice that's become its own kind of disease that gets passed down from one generation of women to the next. I saw it play out recently in real time, on Mother's Day. I was perusing social media and happened upon a video recorded by a man who was praising his wife for being "so selfless." He elaborated at length about how often she goes out of her way to care for him and their children before herself. Expressing his gratitude at length, he repeatedly referred to her as his "hero."

Millions of women watch videos like this every day and share them with friends while oohing and awwing about how "sweet" they are. However, this widespread cultural belief around women needing to be "selfless" is the real problem we're facing.

Truth? That man's "hero" is most likely drowning in her own selflessness. She's likely running herself ragged day after day, physically worn down, emotionally and spiritually depleted, smoldering in pent-up shame, rage, and resentment. She, too, screams at her children more often than she wants to admit and then feels overwhelmed by her own regret and shame. However miserable she may be, she's so convinced that her worth as a mother and human is tied to her "selflessness" that she marches on, day after day, methodically wearing herself down. She does all of this while hiding not just her true desires, but also the fact that she has any at all. Terrified of being found out, she does everything she can to avoid being seen as who she really is.

Why does she do this? Because who she is—at her core, her essence—is a whole human, full of desires. Deep down, she is not so selfless; deep down, she does not embody this essential characteristic of a "good" mother. If she fessed up to being who she really is and having the desires she has had for so long, she would also be revealing herself to be what any "good" mother is *not* supposed to be—an actual person with needs and desires of her own.

Since owning up to her desires would be shameful, she works hard every day to push them down and away, too terrified of what they might mean—that she, at her most basic level, can never be a "good"—as in, selfless—mother. Also, once she truly acknowledges her desires, she will have to face her shame, fear, and other challenging emotions. She will also have to go after what she really wants. What could be more disruptive than a "selfless" woman claiming her right take up space, claim her voice, and achieve her true desires? This "selfless good mother" story is the same one that women have been living since the dawn of time.

In more ways than we may care to admit, this man's "hero" is all of us, playing a role we didn't choose, a role that was assigned to us a long time ago. The widespread, culturally accepted idea that our value as women and mothers lies in our ability to self-sacrifice dates back thousands of years. It's an eternal voice that tells us that our ability to give and give again and then give even more—no matter what all that giving may cost us in terms of our own vitality and fulfillment—is all that truly matters about us.

According to this way of thinking, our worth, as humans, increases the more we self-sacrifice. Yet self-sacrifice means that we die, if not literally, then spiritually and emotionally. It means that there is literally less of us available, both to ourselves and our loved ones. Is that our goal? Is our energetic depletion really what's best for our children? Should they, our offspring, have to watch us wither and die, spiritually or physically, a little more each day? And what does it teach them?

A Time-Honored Tradition

I often ask clients what it felt like watching their own mothers undergo this same process of self-sacrifice. Again and again, they react immediately: "It was awful! I don't want that." Stories of their mothers then pour out—about how they never took care of themselves, about the anger and resentment that came out and was often directed at them when they were children. Over and over again, I hear about their own mothers' battles with depression, anxiety, or extreme dependence, and even mental or emotional incapacity, in their later years.

Too often, they share stories of unabated suffering.

Ironically, every adult daughter of these "selfless" mothers sees the damage it did, yet again and again, to a degree they don't want to admit, many now follow in similar footsteps, valuing others first and themselves last, if at all.

The problem we're facing is not one of personal flaws or individual lack. It is a collective, yet personal pain caused by cultural beliefs that a woman's worth lies in her ability to be selfless and self-sacrificing. Here's how Valerie Rein, PhD, explains this time-honored cultural phenomenon in her book *Patriarchy Stress Disorder*:

> A woman's power has always been a punishable offense. Under patriarchy, it's never been safe for a woman to be visible. For the crime of being visible in their power, women used to be burned at the stake, drowned, and beheaded. We may not have directly been persecuted for our power, but we came from the generations of women before us who have been traumatically conditioned not to reach for the cherry blossoms—because they were either dangerous or unattainable.

(The "cherry blossoms" refer to a study performed on mice, and in this quote symbolize our desires and rewards.)

If we are going to be the mothers and women we have always wanted to be, we have to first recognize this belief, and then be willing to shed it, no matter how scary and uncomfortable that process proves to be.

Recently, after hearing yet another client vent about her husband taking a long dump while she took care of their children, I recorded a podcast episode titled, "I Think It's Time to Take a 40-Minute S#!+"—and I'm serious. Honestly, what's wrong with us, as mothers, taking our time away? Our husbands can take a break. Why can't we?

I ask these questions and so often hear more excuses—about how many people "need" us, about how busy we are, and so on. But let's get serious—will the world really come to an end because you took a forty-minute dump or bath or walk? Routines might change, but will your children really suffer if your husband or neighbor or friend takes over long enough for you to take a break?

Or are you the one who suffers at the thought of taking time for yourself? What do you say to yourself when you're not self-sacrificing? Enough with the excuses already, ladies. What are you really afraid of?

The Gift of Discomfort

Letting yourself be profoundly uncomfortable is one of the greatest gifts you can give yourself. I get that you don't want to. I resisted it so fully and for so long, it took me three children and a cancer diagnosis before I was willing to experience the deep, soul-stirring discomfort of facing myself, feeling my feelings, and reconciling with how often I was self-sacrificing to be a "good" mother.

Alone with my chemo bags and my ailing body, mind, and soul, I was forced to begin facing my shame, my fear, and my anger. Finally, I had to fess up to the big dreams I was dying to realize but petrified to really go for. I was forced to admit that I would never be able to "do it all," and that I'd never forgive myself if I didn't try to make the big impact my soul was aching to make.

Over and over again, I had to let go and feel the many emotions I felt giving my child's day-to-day care to people who *weren't me*. I had to do all of this for months that went on so much longer than I could have imagined as my body slowly, so very slowly, did the monumental healing work it needed to do. It was challenging, but I'm here to tell you that letting yourself be that uncomfortable can be the only way to experience the relief you've long been seeking. Discomfort may unsettle, even rattle you sometimes, but unlike wearing yourself down year after year, discomfort won't kill you.

I'm living proof that we can do this. We can get so sick and tired of giving so much to everyone but ourselves, of feeling perpetually depleted and run down, of hearing ourselves yelling at our children, that finally, we're ready to drop our excuses and feel the discomfort we will feel when we face the reasons we've been self-sacrificing all this time.

Being a Giver

Like you, I am a giver. Even now, when I consistently put myself on my own to-do list, when I make a point of feeling discomfort in order to sense into what I'm really needing and wanting, I remain, at heart, a giver. I give to friends, clients, neighbors. Since the COVID-19 pandemic began, my family and I have been delivering food to people who need it.

When there is need, when there is want, my instinct is to give.

Giving to ourselves does not mean that we stop giving to or caring for others. Here's how I often explain it: Rather than giving away everything we have, let's reverse-engineer this. First, fill your cup. Most women are surprised by how quickly that happens. Depending on how depleted you are, it may take a month or two, or it may take up to a year.

Once your cup is full, whatever comes out of your cup, you give away. Everything that spills out goes to your children, your spouse or partner, your friends, family, community. It all goes to others. But always, you keep your cup full. Always, you give from a full cup.

You remain a giver, but because you're giving from a full cup, your entire experience, your entire life, feels different. You feel replenished, whole, nourished, yet still, you can give away everything you don't need.

Giving Detox

I was talking to a friend and fellow coach who had recently started a new venture around supporting the planet. Unsure what to charge or how to structure her new business, she'd been doing what so many women do—giving her workshops away "by donation."

"Stop with the martyr syndrome," I told her. "You have to stop giving your expertise away."

"But I've been having a hard time receiving," she replied.

"No one's going to knock on your door and give you permission to receive. Put a price on it. Charge real money. When you own your value, you attract people who value you. You have to challenge people to rise up. If you don't, they stay down. You're not helping anyone by not getting paid what you're worth. You're perpetuating a *lack mindset* and supporting the status quo. You say you want to change the world, but your actions aren't energetically aligning with that."

I challenged her to go on a giving detox, start charging for her workshops, and own her value. She accepted immediately, knowing it was time to navigate the discomfort to experience a breakthrough around receiving and claiming her value.

This same principle applies to raising our children. If we model constant self-sacrifice, they expect us to self-sacrifice more and learn that they, too, should grow up and become self-sacrificing. After all, that's what our mothers did, and that's what we're now doing. Why would it be any different for us and our children? However, if we turn it around and model self-nourishment, they learn to do the same for themselves and gain a healthy sense of self.

I'm going to repeat this until it's ingrained in your thinking and way of living: fill your cup first. You can then give away anything that spills out, although you don't have to. Guess what, ladies? You don't just deserve a full cup; you deserve an overflowing one! Sometimes you can give away the extra; sometimes you can keep it for yourself. You get to decide.

If that feels like a new concept, you will have to navigate discomfort in order to practice this. None of it will feel natural or justified at first, and you may finally have to experience the emotions—shame, fear, regret, guilt, anger, and more—that you've been afraid of feeling. However, if you continue practicing filling your cup first, you, too, can experience profound transformations.

When Sara began living this way, her energy completely changed. As a working mother of four children, with a full-time job, new side business, and a husband who traveled often for his job, she'd been defaulting to her excuses around money, time, her children, and her energy for years. Once we were working together and she began to focus on filling her cup first, she realized that she could, in fact, take a twenty-minute walk in the woods near her house on a busy day. She could also take a few minutes to journal, self-reflect, and get centered. She could even take an occasional break from social media without sabotaging her business. She could do all of this while being a parent, employee, and wife and feel more energized, expansive, and flexible precisely because she was filling her own cup first.

Parenting Is Not a Roadblock

Filling your cup begins with figuring out what you want. When I first ask clients what they want, they often reply with one of two things. The first, and most common, is, "I don't know what I want."

We've already talked about "I don't know" being an excuse, as well as a lie. Deep down, we know what we want. We know how we want to feel and how we want to live. We use "I don't know" to avoid facing our true desires. We do this because facing our desires means facing the shame of being a woman and having desires, which, as we've seen, is still taboo—an admission that we're not, in fact, as "selfless" as a "good" mother should be.

The other reply I hear most often is, "I'll go after my dreams once I fix my parenting."

Women say this in all kinds of ways, but the essence is, they need to feel worthy as a mother before they feel like they're "allowed" to go after their dreams. Again, this supports the idea that as good mothers, we should be operating from an empty cup.

Selflessness doesn't serve anyone, including—especially—our children. Think back on your own "selfless" mother, if you had one, and be honest about how that impacted you as a child. Was she angry, impatient, depressed? Even if you're not exhibiting her same attitudes and behaviors, is your self-lessness really serving your children? Or is your exhaustion, depletion, and resulting anger and impatience detracting from their lives?

We need to stop using parenting and our children as a road-block. Our children are not the reason we're not taking action to realize our dreams and desires. They are not to blame for us not going for what we want. Only you can stop yourself from going after what you want. That process begins with figuring out your Big Why.

Finding Your Big Why

Why are you here? What drew you to me and this book?

Most likely, you are embarking on a spiritual, mental, emotional, and physical journey similar to the one I embraced when I was diagnosed with cancer. Honestly? Some days are going to suck. Some days you're going to want to give up, and that's when you'll really need your Big Why.

Simon Sinek, author of *Find Your Why*, explains it this way: "We don't necessarily find happiness in our jobs every day, but we can feel fulfilled by our work every day if it makes us feel part of something bigger than ourselves."

Life will never be all rainbows and sunshine, but we can feel like our efforts are worthwhile when they're connected to a bigger purpose, which is what I call your Big Why. That Big Why keeps you focused on moving forward in this journey every day, even when you don't want to, even when you feel guilty about investing time in your dreams, even when you can't spend money or time, even when you [fill in the excuse], even when you [fill in the excuse], and on and on.

Your Big Why is your reason for persevering. Figuring out your Big Why is actually pretty simple. It's a five-minute exercise you can do with nothing more than your journal, a pen, and an open mind. Are you ready?

This is a freewriting exercise, so don't overthink things. Just write down any thoughts that come to mind. To begin, open to a blank page in your journal. Set a five-minute timer on your phone. At the top of your page, write, *What do I want?*

It doesn't matter how big or small your "wants" are. Just write them down as they come to you.

I want to stop yelling.
I want to make more money.
I want peace and quiet.
I want to spend less time in the car.

I want to quit my job.

I want financial freedom.

I want to lose ten pounds.

Once you have a list, go to the want on your list that most speaks to you at this moment.

For example, let's say it's "I want to make more money." Ask yourself why you want to make more money. Write down your answer.

I want to feel free and calm.

Again, ask yourself why: Why do I want to feel free and calm?

Because I want to feel good.

Again, why?

Because there's so much I want to do.

Again, why?

Because the planet is dying, and I want to help heal it so my children and grandchildren can live healthy, fulfilling lives.

Keep asking why until you get to an answer that feels like a core Big Why—the deeper reason you're motivated to show up, even when life feels hard.

Once you've gotten to something that feels like your Big Why, write it somewhere you will see it every day. This isn't set in stone; know that you can always update or change it. As always, we're focusing on progress, so don't wait to find the "perfect" Big Why. Drill down to something and go with that for now.

A Reminder about Journaling

If you're like one of the many women I've met who resist journaling, I get it, but I'm going to invite you to use it as a tool anyway. I've worked with so many clients who initially say they don't like it or don't find it useful, only to end up loving it. When you don't worry about journaling the "right way," it's an incredibly powerful way to tap into your intuition and trust what it's telling you.

As women, we hold more answers inside us than we consciously acknowledge. In order to tap into that knowing, we have to take action. Journaling is a great initial action step to take, so, please, do not skip this step! If you only sit around thinking about advancing your spiritual journey, you're not making any actual progress. You must match your intention with action.

Now that you've got your Big Why, it's time to begin creating your new lifestyle plan.

Creating Your Starter Lifestyle Plan

You know when you're daydreaming and it's so clear what you want? What do you envision? Do you see yourself on a beach with no one to watch over and nothing you have to do? Or feeling fabulous as you get ready for a fun night out? Or reading a book uninterrupted?

Let yourself dream for a moment. Try to let go of all your limitations, to-dos and have-tos, and just dream. What comes to mind?

If any of your answers were about other people doing and not doing something, bring it back to yourself and let yourself actually dream. For instance, if you told yourself that you wanted your children to have fewer tantrums or do homework without you having to nag them constantly, that's not a dream; it's something you want less of in your life. Really try to focus on what *you want*. If focusing on yourself in this way feels uncomfortable, that's an indication that this is exactly what you need to be doing. If you feel too much discomfort, or resistance, to think of anything, do some freewriting in your journal starting with this prompt:

It's too uncomfortable for me to focus on just myself because...

When we talk about desires and goals, we of course have to return to how we want to feel.

Every time we think about achieving a goal, we're actually envisioning how we think we'll *feel* once we've achieved it. For example, losing ten pounds might actually be about wanting to feel comfortable in your own skin. Similarly, making more money might be about wanting to feel free. It's always the feeling we're seeking; the goal is a way to feel that feeling.

Focusing on how you want to feel doesn't necessarily mean that you overlook the goal itself. You can lose ten pounds and make more money, but by focusing first on how you want to feel, you not only connect to yourself more deeply, you also ground yourself in your desires, which makes it easier to manifest what you desire.

Let's get started. Get your journal and keep it on hand. Find a comfortable, quiet spot and read through these lists, letting yourself really feel into the emotions you want to embody. Keep in mind, these lists only include a small number of the many emotions we may feel, so don't hesitate to write emotions that don't appear below.

Depressed	Angry	Sad	Afraid	Hurt
Disappointed	Irritated	Lonely	Fearful	Pained
Pessimistic	Frustrated	Dismayed	Anxious	Rejected
Powerless	Resentful	Blindsided	Rigid	Humiliated
Alienated	Controlling	Oversensitive	Prejudiced	Wronged
Stuck	Agitated	Tearful	Self-conscious	Secretive
Resistant	Short-tempered	Unworthy	Defensive	Deprived

Open	Loving	Happy	Alive	Positive
Confident	Compassionate	Thankful	Playful	Hopeful
Understanding	Considerate	Fun-loving	Courageous	Creative
Receptive	Affectionate	Mellow	Optimistic	Motivated
Flexible	Appreciative	Joyous	Giving	Adaptable
Friendly	Respectful	Festive	Excited	Brave

After reading through the lists as many times as you need to, write down the five feelings you most want to feel. These are the foundation of your lifestyle plan.

Associating Desires with Actions

Now it's time to consider action. You'll hear me talk about taking action, specifically courageous action, a lot. You won't experience desired changes if you're not taking action in your life. Manifesting requires intention + action. If you forgo taking action, you won't create what you desire.

Taking action can feel scary, I know, but it's a critical part of the process. Don't wait until you don't feel scared to take action; that day will never come. You have to feel the fear and take action anyway. That's what I did every day when my life was on the line. I focused on living, even though I was terrified. You can do it too.

To begin, turn to a blank page in your journal and draw a line straight down the middle. Label the left column *How I want to feel*, and the right column *Action*.

At the top of the feelings column, write down your first desired emotion. In the action column, write down the actions you can take to feel that way. For example:

How I want to feel	Action
Connected	Meet friend for coffee
	Cook with family
	Backyard picnic with neighbors
	Weekly date night
	Meditate each morning (to connect to myself)

Add another four ways you want to feel to your page, writing in actions for each. Don't worry about how many actions are on your list. This is about noticing what types of actions you can take to feel how you want to feel.

The Creative Process of Determining Your Desires

How are you feeling? Do your desired feelings seem authentic and inspiring? So often, clients begin with one set of feelings and realize over time that their original list isn't as on point as they originally thought it was. This often happens after they begin taking action and realize they still aren't feeling how they want to feel.

Homing in on your desired feelings and the actions you can take to experience them is a creative process. Your lists of desired feelings and actions can and should evolve over time. Instead of wanting to feel fulfilled, you may realize that what you're actually seeking is the feeling of being inspired. Similarly, an action such as going to yoga class may have once felt inspiring but doesn't right now. Let yourself notice and adapt to these natural ebbs and flows. Change your desired feelings and actions according to how you want to feel at different times.

End of Chapter Exercise: Take Action!

I love feeling challenged, and nothing does that quite like taking action. Now it's your turn! For three days, take at least one action per day on your top three desired feelings.

At the end of each day, jot down observations in your journal so you have a log of how and when your actions have or haven't helped you to feel your desired feelings.

12

Energetic Time Management

WHAT CAN I DO *right now to feel strong and alive?*
While undergoing chemo, I wanted to feel *strong* and *alive,* so I asked myself that question over and over again, day after day.

As my weeks of chemo turned into months of recovery, I began to dig deeper into the process, determined to bring my desired feelings to life as much and as often as I could. Before long, I realized that time management wasn't enough—I had to have the energy I needed too.

Determined to make the most of my time and energy, I slowly but surely created a system I now call Energetic Time Management (ETM). It started with one talk, then grew over time. Once I got the hang of it, it changed so much about how I scheduled my time and "spent" my energy that I began teaching it to clients. By now, it's revolutionized how thousands of clients approach their daily lives. Instead of feeling imprisoned by their schedules or energy, they now know that they can harness both to change how they feel.

When was the last time you went through a day or week feeling how you wanted to feel? When was the last time you made feeling that way more important than completing more tasks? Now that you're becoming aware of your excuses, it's time to make a deep and lasting commitment to your desired feelings and use them to reinvent how you navigate your days.

Task Mastering Is *Not* Living

Marty had been in my coaching program for months when she reached out to me. Her voice and energy seemed off. When I asked her what was happening, she started talking about productivity and her desired feelings. "I'm a good taskmaster," she began. "I feel like my desired feelings are genuinely what I want, but then I look at my calendar and I have things like cleaning my car scheduled for Saturday."

I see this so often—women zeroing in on how they want to feel only to resort to showing up, yet again, as the taskmasters they're used to being. In fact, a few days before speaking with Marty, another woman had made a similar comment after an online talk I'd given about ETM: "I struggle with perfectionism and letting others dictate my schedule. I feel like I never have enough time."

So many women I've met are incredibly good at getting things done. They excel at their jobs, run their household, and do as much as they can to stay on top of their children's homework, social and activity calendars, healthcare, and social/emotional well-being. While they may not achieve every result they desire, they try really, really hard.

When I ask them to put some of their time and energy into making themselves a priority, at first, they seem receptive, even motivated, to finally give back to themselves. But then they soon return to what they know—scheduling and ticking off tasks that bring them zero joy and have nothing to do with how *they* want to feel.

Why is this "get more done" mentality so hard for us to overcome?

We've all been programmed to manage time, which we've been told means accomplishing as many tasks as we can. This, we've been taught to believe, is what will make us "successful." Wanting to succeed, we're forever trying to squeeze in one more thing, and then another after that. That's what accomplished people do, isn't it?

Month after month, year after year, we strive and seek, always accomplishing more for everyone and everything around us. Eventually, we exhaust ourselves to the point where even our accomplishments feel meaningless. In the midst of all of our doing, we lose ourselves and our joy too.

Instead of always seeking to do more, we need to learn to give ourselves permission to matter; to fill our cups first and recognize that doing this is, unto itself, a way of giving to ourselves *and* to those who love us and rely on us. Remember, when our cup is filled first, we have more of what truly matters— joy, love, connection—to give. With ETM, we can put this idea into practice every day.

As we dive deeper into this work, let me be clear—ETM is *not* a calendaring system. It is *not* a new form of list making. It sometimes involves both of those activities, but really, it's about making profound shifts in how you feel about yourself, your life, and how you live every day. This is not a "one and done" system or a "set it and forget it" formula. It's a practice that you'll have to implement each day. Some days it will come more easily. Some days it may feel more challenging. However, as I've seen with myself and so many of my clients, once you truly commit to transforming your life with ETM, your desired feelings begin to come alive inside you.

Which Desires Are Really Running Your Day?

You know how you want to feel, but what's motivating your actions?

When I asked Marty why she was continuing to schedule tasks like cleaning her car during her free time, she said that she was worried someone would see her messy car and judge her for it. Not being judged had nothing to do with how she wanted to feel, but other people's judgments were still a stronger determinant in how she was spending her time and energy than her desired feelings were.

Another client realized that she felt resentful toward her boss because she hadn't been respecting herself or her own time and energy when it came to his needs. Instead, she'd been allowing him to dictate how she spent her time and energy at work, as well as on weekends and holidays. Like Marty, she'd been overlooking her desired feelings and allowing her time and energy to be used by others on their terms, not hers.

Our time and energy are our most precious resources. Why are we giving them away so easily? Why does the woman who commented after my ETM talk regularly let other people schedule *her* time according to *their* priorities?

Even once we've reached executive positions, even once our children have grown more independent, even once we've had ample coaching and done years of personal development work, we're still defaulting to a habit that's so deeply ingrained in us, we hardly notice it.

That habit is people-pleasing.

Over and over again, we do for others before we do for ourselves. The moment we're "needed" or "wanted," we abandon our own needs and desires in order to give to our children, spouse or partner, friend, colleague, family—even total strangers. What's it going to take for us to start putting ourselves and our respect for our own bodies, minds, and souls on the front burner?

In spite of what we've been conditioned to believe, being a nurturer does not require self-sacrifice. Being a "good" mother—or employee, friend, daughter, neighbor, boss, and more—does not mean valuing others above ourselves. We can value ourselves *and* care for others. We can give to ourselves and *then* give to others. We can nurture from a full cup. Why do we resist that idea so much that we hesitate to even try? Why do we spend valuable time and money doing personal development work only to rush back to our people-pleasing behaviors?

Zeroing in on our desired feelings is an important first step in this journey, but when you begin practicing ETM, you invariably discover where your true challenges lie. This is what I mean when I say that ETM isn't a calendaring system or a "set it and forget it" formula. We're not cooking a rotisserie chicken, ladies! It's something you have to show up for and practice every single day. Most of us literally have to learn how to value ourselves from the ground up—the way we did when we were much younger, the way we did before the world told us we had to self-sacrifice and people-please in order to be judged as "good" by the world.

Setting Boundaries

You've no doubt spent years waiting for "things" to change. But then time passes, you get more help, the kids grow older, you get promoted, hire an assistant, and move to a new house— all kinds of once-desired external changes happen—and still, your time and energy do not feel like your own.

And you know what? You're right. Your time and energy still aren't your own because you're still giving them away. By not taking a stand for your needs and your desires and not setting boundaries, you're allowing others to assume control of your time and energy. You're waiting for others to give you permission to value yourself when the only person's permission you need is your own.

Think about that for a minute. You can never get today back, and there's only so much energy you can "spend" before you need sleep. Your time and energy are your most precious resources, yet still, you're letting others decide how, when, where, and why they're used. This is a perfect way to feel out of control.

So why are we still doing this? Why are we still saying yes— to volunteer opportunities, social gatherings, and more—that are killing us one day at a time, one decision at a time? Unless and until we actively and proactively claim our time and energy as our own, they *will* belong to others. In order to take control of our own time and energy, we have to set boundaries. We have to stop saying yes to people, places, and things that consume our time and energy but bring us no closer to our desires.

We are powerful, amazing creatures who do so much and willingly take charge in so many ways. Why are we so afraid of saying such a tiny, two-letter word: "no"?

When we operate from this place and say yes to people and things that deplete us and take us away from how we want to feel, we are operating from a place of lack. The actions we take validate our feelings of not being enough. Every time we say yes when we mean no, we are telling ourselves that our own needs and desires don't matter, that we don't even deserve our own time and energy.

By establishing healthy boundaries, we move away from lack and toward abundance. We give our desired feelings and outcomes time and space to grow.

Since the early days of my working from home, I've had to set very clear boundaries, even with people I sincerely love spending time with. At one point, knowing that I was home, friends and neighbors began stopping by unannounced. Knowing that I needed to focus on realizing my big career dreams, I had to let people know that I couldn't accommodate unplanned midday drop-ins. It wasn't always easy. Were these unplanned visits an easy distraction from working? *Yes!* But I had to feel my discomfort and create space to get things done. Were people offended? Maybe at first. I honestly don't know. What I do know is that creating that space to focus on my work has allowed me to build a seven-figure business that has been an ongoing source of fulfillment and abundance. Whatever awkwardness may have briefly existed has long since dissipated, allowing me to nurture my desires and my friendships, just at separate times during the week.

"No" and "I can't today" and "not right now" are powerful words. So much good can come from allowing our desires to become real priorities in our daily lives. We need to work through the discomfort of saying those words, step into our brave zones, and say them often and out loud so we can finally feel the feelings and live the life we desire.

Saying no isn't about us, and it is *not* a way of being selfish. Even when people don't want to hear no, it often serves them, as well as us. Instead of enabling their dependence, for example, it might push them to step into their own brave zone and feel more of how they want to feel.

Finding Your Energy Leaks

We all have energy leaks—places inside us that seep precious energy that we need in order to live and thrive. They are areas we need to patch, but often those leaks feel like they're coming from outside of us, from somewhere or something we try to control but fail to. The first step in patching those leaks is identifying them.

With that idea in mind, take out your journal and write down all of the people and things that are sucking the life out of you. Write freely and honestly, without judgment. This list is for your eyes only, so if a child's behavior or your messy house or money stress—or all three of those and much more—are depleting you, write them all down.

While you may not yet know how to patch these leaks, they are inside you. They are yours and you *can* control them. We'll look at how to do that in detail later, but for now all you need to do is recognize where they are. Keep your list for later reference.

Using Resentment as a Guide

We've been so programmed to say yes and accommodate others' needs before our own that we don't always know where our boundaries actually lie. To figure that out, start noticing when, why, and with whom you tend to feel angry or resentful. If you're feeling resentful at work, start noticing when you're saying yes but would like to say no. If you're feeling resentful at home, notice what's happening that's making you feel that way. Then ask yourself what kind of boundary you can set to address the issue. For example, let's say you feel guilty about working all day. When your children's bedtime arrives, you let it slip, telling yourself you "owe" them that extra time. Before long, they're overtired and hyperactive, and you're exhausted and fed up. What could have been an enjoyable on-time bedtime turns into yelling in order to (finally) get them into bed. By the time you're finally able to get to bed yourself, you're seething with resentment. That's a good indication that bed-time needs better boundaries. By prioritizing sleep for you and your children, you will all feel better and enjoy what time you do have together more.

Setting boundaries is a process and not something that comes naturally to a lot of us. This is the kind of work that's most effective with close friend or a coach who will call you out when you're not following through. Saying no and establishing healthy boundaries may not feel easy, especially at first, but you can't implement the nuts and bolts of ETM without first doing this.

Before we discuss how ETM works, we need to address another idea that tends to distract us from our desired feelings. That idea is balance, or as I like to call it, the b-word.

Are We Seeking Balance or Alignment?

Oh, here it comes... I can feel it. The interviewer is setting up the question. My blood pressure is rising. My lips are sealed. I want to scream but I don't; that's not professional.

Ugh, I think I can smell dog poop from the other room, but I can't clean it up because I'm being interviewed on Zoom for someone's podcast. I mute myself as one of the boys tells the other one to fuck off.

"Tell us, how do you fit it all in?" she finally asks me.

I know what she's waiting for. I know she wants to hear about the b-word. She and her audience are hoping I'll reveal some secret about how I "balance it all"—which also means I'm about to disappoint everyone.

Honestly? I don't balance it all. I don't even *try* to balance it all.

What does the question *How do you fit all in?* even mean? And why do I even have to answer it or even write about it?

Men aren't asked this question. They are human, like us, but it's okay for them. We don't judge them for what they *don't do*, only for what they *do*.

For women, it's different. Women are expected to do it all, and in turn, we expect ourselves to do it all.

Is this interviewer actually asking me how I overload my plate with unrealistic expectations and, in the process, asking me to validate unrealistic expectations around what being a "good" mother and woman means?

How does our stretching ourselves to the breaking point make us more caring mothers, not to mention healthy, fulfilled humans? This whole idea that we should be "doing it all" is poison. It's a trick and we're all falling for it, day after day, year after year.

So, to answer the question, no, I don't "do it all" and I can't always "make it all work." From one hour and one day to the next, my life, like yours, is constantly changing. At any given time, different parts of my life are expanding and contracting in unequal and unpredictable ways. At no time do the many parts of my life fit into proportionate time slots or energy buckets. Sometimes my boys need more of my time and energy. Sometimes it's my business, travel, or physical well-being. More often, several different parts of my life are expanding in opposing directions at once. If my goal was balance, I'd be setting myself up for continual failure. Instead, I constantly return to a different question: *What do I need?*

The question we should be asking is, *Why are we so enchanted by the idea of balance?* Why has living a "balanced life" taken hold of our collective consciousness?

Based on what I've experienced and heard from clients and followers for years, we've been collectively brainwashed into believing that living a so-called balanced life will allow us to feel peaceful, calm, and contented; or joyful, inspired, and loved, and so on. Whatever ways we want to feel will happen once our lives are "balanced"—or so we've been told and keep telling ourselves. Tell me something, though, do any of the women you know well have a balanced life?

Probably not, and that's because we're not actually seeking balance. We're yearning to feel how we think balance will allow us to feel. We're desperately seeking our desired feelings.

The Secret Ingredient to Creating Change

Even once we know we're yearning to feel certain ways, we put our time and energy into setting accomplishment-based goals and achieving the ever-elusive "balanced life." Year after year, we commit to doing our personal development work, yet put most of our focus on adjusting the various parts of our *external* lives.

If that method worked, wouldn't you already feel how you want to feel? Think about all of the big dreams you've already achieved—did you get married? Build a career? Get promoted? Have children? Buy a house? Travel? Think back on what you were yearning to achieve years ago. You may be surprised by the number of external changes you've successfully realized.

So, what happened? When you became a mother, did you feel how you envisioned you would? When you got the job or the promotion, when you bought the house or lost those five pounds, did you feel how you wanted to feel? And if so, did those feelings last, or were they relatively fleeting?

If external change could create lasting internal change, wouldn't you already feel peaceful, calm, and contented, or however you want to feel? If you're not closer to your desired feelings, it's because external life changes can't change your internal life. When clients tell me they want more space, they usually don't need a bigger house. Occupying more square footage will give them more to take care of and may even increase feelings of loneliness. Instead of more physical space, they're in fact seeking a feeling of spaciousness. In many cases, they find the space they're seeking by creating their own. Taking a solo walk or long solitary drive, enjoying a bath with the door locked, or implementing a meditation or yoga practice—all of these actions can help you to feel spacious, especially when they're repeated on a regular basis.

External changes *do not* and *cannot* create lasting internal change. We know this, but still we work diligently to pretend that we don't. To really change our lives, to truly ditch self-sacrifice and step into our brave zone, we have to show up and do the internal work.

As we move into the practice of Energetic Time Management, it's really important to remember that ETM won't bring you closer to your desired feelings if you're not doing the internal work. True and lasting transformative change only happens from the inside out.

Showing Up—Even When It's Imperfect

For the second day in a row, I'd forgotten I had an online meeting with my book writer/co-creator. By the time I realized what I'd done—call it pandemic brain fog—I was parked at Starbucks just after picking up my drive-through order. About to head home, I decided to stay put instead and grabbed my phone to join the meeting. As we started talking, I began voicing how I was feeling in the midst of our collective turmoil and uncertainty. After a while, we got to work and ended up going over our scheduled time by almost half an hour.

Since I was already overscheduled that day, that extra half hour was arguably time I didn't have to spare. However, that "wasted" half hour had also helped me feel a little lighter; it had helped me to fill my cup. Rather than stressing over how much I had to do after the meeting, I allowed myself to enjoy that little bit of relief.

That's one of the countless examples of how I practice ETM every day. It's never a perfect formula, and I rarely accomplish every single task on my to-do list for the day. However, I do typically accomplish my highest priority tasks while also allowing myself opportunities—some planned, some not—to feel more of how I want to feel. As long as I show up and do whatever I can—however imperfectly—to manifest my desired feelings, I know I'm moving forward in my spiritual journey and my life.

Choosing Imperfection over All-or-Nothing

Stories like these are important because they highlight an issue many of my clients run into when they begin practicing ETM. Because most of us are accustomed to being taskmasters—to planning time without considering energy or emotions—they tend to approach ETM first and foremost as a scheduling system. As a result, especially at first, they make ETM about what they do each day rather than how they feel. They then assess their progress with an all-or-nothing mindset.

When we approach ETM this way, we not only distort it by avoiding the inner work and turning it into a time management system, we also invalidate the small but important internal shifts that can eventually add up to significant, lasting inner transformation.

To put this into concrete terms, here's an example: Let's say you commit to doing five minutes of meditation each day in order to feel more peaceful. Over a period of days or weeks, you then start to feel a little less stressed. There's no enormous change or result you can pinpoint, but you do feel a little better. With an all-or-nothing mindset, that little improvement in how you feel quickly loses its value because you don't feel *completely* different or *all* better. According to that way of thinking, you'd be better off skipping meditation and spending Saturday cleaning the car. At least then, at the end of that day, you'd clearly see a difference and feel a sense of accomplishment. However, that feeling of having achieved something worthwhile doesn't last because a few minutes after finishing your car, the children start fighting, you start yelling, and your newly cleaned car is no longer giving you the feeling of peace you yearn for.

I can't say this enough—ETM, and all of your spiritual journey, is about progress, not perfection. I don't practice ETM perfectly. In fact, accepting your imperfections is part of ETM. Allowing yourself to feel better, even when nothing about you or your life is perfect, is part of the journey. If those five minutes of meditation help you to feel a little more of your desired feelings, then it should remain a priority! Remember, ETM may change how you navigate your days, but it's mostly about showing up for the inner work that will allow you to feel your desired feelings.

Putting ETM to Work in Your Daily Life

To set up ETM from scratch, you will need to complete six steps. Since your attention goes wherever your energy goes, I recommend carving out two hours and a quiet space where you can give this process your focused thought and attention.

Go to dyingtobeagoodmother.com to download the ETM Worksheet, a step-by-step process to manage your energy, not your time.

Step 1: The Brain Dump

The first step for setting up ETM is the brain dump.

We all have an endless list of to-dos. They may not fill our soul, but they can fill long stretches of time and mental space, if we let them. Before looking at what you desire, you need to clear out that mental clutter.

You'll do that next by making a brain dump list. This is where you purge your should-dos, need-to-dos, have-to-dos, even your want-to-dos. Put it all down so you can eliminate your feelings of overwhelm.

When I do this, I break my list down by these categories:

- Self
- Kids
- Relationships
- Money
- Work
- Physical environment
- Other

You don't have to brain dump for every category. Your goal is just to get all of your to-dos on the page. You can also write a list without categories and sort them into categories later.

On a blank journal page, do your brain dump. Purge onto the page so you can at least clear out the mental space you'll need to move forward.

Step 2: Prioritize

I know it's tempting to start burning through the list you just made. Please don't do that! To move toward your desired feelings and your big vision, you have to prioritize your list. This isn't necessarily about doing what feels good in the moment. It's about giving your time and energy to tasks that move you toward your desires. That will mean being uncomfortable at times. In fact, you may have already experienced discomfort when I asked you not to burn through the tasks on your brain dump list. The truth is, being busy and staying busy is easy. What's not always easy is saying no to your old priorities in order to say yes to creating the life you desire.

With that in mind, next you're going to prioritize your life. You should always be number one on that list; fueling yourself first will allow you to manifest your desired feelings, realize your bigger vision, and show up as your best self. Here's a sample priority list:

1. Self
2. Money
3. My kids
4. My partner or spouse
5. My house
6. Friends
7. Volunteer work

Below your prioritized list, write down your top three desired feelings. If you're feeling overwhelmed, remember that this is a process. You can write down one or two desired feelings. You're not going to master ETM in one day or even one week, and that's okay. We're taking baby steps. Each baby step counts as progress. All you need to do is show up and do what you can.

Step 3: Highest Leveraged Action
Now you'll begin to make space for actions that align with your desired feelings.

Don't worry if ETM is still a little unclear. As you continue using this system week after week, you'll be waking up to yourself and figuring out how to continue creating the life you desire. If you're working on mastering the basics—exercising, getting sleep, drinking water, and so on—then focus on those for a while. Remember, though, we're moving away from all-or-nothing thinking. Instead, aim to improve your habits and how you feel by one degree. For example, don't try to go from drinking no water to four liters a day. Instead, drink one glass of water every morning to start. Focus on improvement, not perfection.

Next, under each of the categories in your brain dump list, write down one to three action steps.

For example, it really helps me to get dressed every morning and do my hair. It elevates my energy and makes me feel better about myself. Mindfulness and exercise also help me to feel mentally and physically vibrant and ready for whatever my day brings. If my desired feelings are confident, strong, and alive, my action list for my "Self" item might look like this:

a. Daily movement for twenty minutes (yoga, running, walking, or gym)
b. Get dressed and do my hair
c. Practice some form of mindfulness for five minutes

Complete this process for each category, always focusing on actions that help you manifest your desired feelings. Remember, this is not a to-do list. Of course, doing laundry and grocery shopping are tasks that need to happen, but because they won't bring you closer to your desired feelings, they shouldn't appear on these lists. However, dancing and singing in your living room might, for example, make you feel sexy or powerful or whatever you want to feel. If the action aligns with a desired feeling, it should appear on your ETM action list, especially as you develop more life-enhancing habits.

Step 4: Set Up Your Calendars

Now it's time to begin putting your vision into action.

At this stage in the process, I highly recommend getting a paper planner instead of just a digital one. There's something that happens with pen and paper that doesn't happen with digital—we relax, access different parts of the brain, and get more creative. That doesn't mean you shouldn't add events to a digital calendar. It just means that it's best for you to also use a paper planner. I use a planner that breaks each day down hourly. That level of planning used to turn me off, but now I prefer it because it helps me to use my time more intentionally.

So often, when we're scheduling our days, we pack in more than we can reasonably handle and then feel overwhelmed because we're "so busy." In reality, we're just not planning effectively. Here's an example I see often: You start scheduling your day by adding your in-person meeting (10 to 11 a.m.) and your child's 4:45 p.m. sports game, since those both occur at fixed times. Then you start adding your ETM actions, followed by work tasks and calls, et cetera. Everything seems to fit into your day, but only on paper, because you've neglected to factor in the time it will take to drive to and from the meeting, as well as your driving time to and from your child's game. That forgotten time accounts for over ninety minutes that you haven't factored into your plans. As a result, before you've even begun your day, you're ninety-plus minutes behind schedule simply because you haven't put enough thought into your planning. For that reason, it's important to take time to sit somewhere uninterrupted and carefully consider how your day will flow.

Another issue that tends to overwhelm is our tendency to try to squeeze in extra tasks, calls, and appointments. For example, when someone asks you to join a call at the last minute, do you say yes, telling yourself that you'll use a Bluetooth headset and run errands while you're on the call? It's tempting, I know, but when that becomes a habit, we end up feeling rushed all day every day. Instead of saying yes to that last-minute invitation or call, start saying no. Non-essential additions often add to feelings of overwhelm and take you further away from your desired feelings. Start noticing events and tasks that are out of alignment with your desired feelings and set healthier boundaries around your time and energy.

The first items you should add to your calendar are the top one to three "Self" category action steps you created in the Highest Leveraged Action step (Step 3) of this process. If putting yourself on your calendar is new for you, this may feel uncomfortable. Again, this is a process that you'll refine over time, but go ahead and write those top actions in the "Self" category into your schedule first. In my case, that means adding showering and doing my hair to my calendar. I have to create space for that. Otherwise, I'll convince myself I don't have the time, and it won't happen. Nothing is too simple to plan for, so whatever you can do to move toward your desired feelings should be added to a time slot in your calendar.

Once you've added your top actions from your "Self" category action list to your calendar, fill in any appointments or events, being sure to factor in prep time, driving time, et cetera. You can try doing this one day at a time or plan an entire week all at once.

Step 5: Taking Action

Putting your plan into action is where the magic happens. If you're setting yourself up for success, you'll make micro-adjustments from one week to the next. Remember, incremental improvement is your goal. Please don't try to make enormous changes right away. I'd much rather you show up for 10 percent of your big plan than get so overwhelmed by aiming for 100 percent that you make no progress. The only thing I call failure is quitting, so doing 10 percent, or even 1 percent, is still success.

Go through your day, doing what you can to adhere to your schedule.

Step 6: Nightly Check-In

Just getting to this point is a milestone unto itself! This last step is important, but also something most people avoid, especially at first. That resistance is normal, and seeing it for what it is—resistance, not failure—is a huge part of your personal development journey. As you practice ETM, life, as well as your emotions, will get in the way. That's normal. This is a process, and again, your focus needs to be on progress, not perfection.

Every night I want you to look at your calendar and take a minute to consider what's happening tomorrow. I like to visualize things involved in our morning routine: *Do we have breakfast food in the house? Will one of my kids freak out about socks? Have I prepped my food yet?* I also visualize my workday: *Is there anyone I need to communicate with? Are there any specific deliverables I need to complete?* Nothing is too mundane or complex. Just try to picture what might happen tomorrow and, when possible, go do a little prep—for example, find socks for your child or take a quick inventory of your pantry. You don't have to "do it all" before bedtime. Just get grounded in what's coming up so you can prepare mentally and logistically.

THAT'S ETM in a nutshell! The more you practice it, the more you'll notice where you experience resistance and how that resistance shows up. One way that commonly occurs is through the stories we tell ourselves about what we "should" do and how we "should" be. In the next chapter we'll look at how we limit ourselves with these stories and also look at how changing them can allow us to experience our desired feelings.

Energetic Time Management (ETM) Recap and Reminders

In addition to staying open to adjusting your Big Why and creating systems and routines that support your ability to take courageous action, it's important to be committed and flexible with how you practice ETM.

To keep yourself moving toward your bigger vision, it is essential to be consistent about practicing ETM. However, your practice can and should change as you and your life evolve. Keep in mind that what worked for you last week, last month, or last year may not fit now. Remember, ETM is not a scheduling or time-management system. Nor is it a one-and-done solution. It's an ongoing practice that consists of these six basic steps:

Step 1: Defining your Big Why—your reason for being on this journey in the first place

Step 2: Creating your bigger vision—of the life you most desire to live

Step 3: Identifying how you want to feel (your desired feelings)

Step 4: Aligning how you spend your time and energy with your desires (practicing ETM daily)

Step 5: Taking courageous action (implementing ETM daily)

Step 6: Navigating the big emotions, aka resistance, that arise as you practice ETM

13

Unearthing Limiting Beliefs and Feeling Big Emotions

BEING A GOOD MOTHER *means self-sacrificing all parts of yourself.*

That was the story I told myself for years. It was also the story that dictated my actions and reactions. Like my clients and probably like many of you, I didn't speak those words out loud. I didn't wake up in the morning and ask how much of myself I would sacrifice that day. Nor did I necessarily wake up and wonder how I could become a better mother. However, when I was (finally) heading out the door to attend a yoga class for the first time in months and one of my children would ask me to play Legos, I would stuff down my despair, say yes, and skip (yet another) class.

What never occurred to me was that I could go to yoga *and* play Legos, just not at the same time. What never crossed my mind was that taking care of myself first would make me a more attentive and mentally and emotionally available mother.

If I'd gone to those yoga classes, I would have returned feeling refreshed, renewed, even excited to spend some quality time with my kids. Instead, I told myself that whatever I was doing for my children wasn't enough; that they needed me, that I had to be there exactly when they needed me, regardless of how it was affecting my health and well-being.

While I was often available, I was also physically, mentally, and emotionally worn down. I also resented "having to" feel that way. For years I was so committed to the story that motherhood required self-sacrifice that all I had left to give my children was a shadow of my actual self.

I am grateful for what cancer forced me to see about myself and my life, but let me be clear—I came very, very close to dying. Continually abandoning myself was *not* worth it. While I don't blame myself for my cancer, I do take personal responsibility for turning a blind eye to my health. I almost lost the only thing that matters—time. My long-standing commitment to the story that motherhood required me to meet everyone's needs except my own almost robbed three amazing boys of their mother. By not taking care of myself, I was being selfish, not selfless; I was using motherhood to avoid facing my intense discomfort around my own worthiness. It was easier to believe that I didn't deserve my own time or TLC. It was easier to self-sacrifice than to take a long and honest look in the mirror and face the rage, shame, and fear that had haunted me since childhood.

Thankfully, I'm still here; my boys still have their mother. Unlike so many mothers who are taken too soon, I have been granted the opportunity to face my own self-limiting beliefs and accept the lifelong challenge of feeling my big emotions and continuously rewriting what it means to be a mother and a woman—to be me.

Since you're reading this, now it's your turn. As you identify your desired feelings and practice ETM, you and countless other women and mothers like you can do the sometimes exhilarating, sometimes exhausting and terrifying work of facing your old stories and writing new and more empowering ones. Let's look at that process in more depth.

Beliefs That Seem Like the Truth

As you integrate ETM into your life on a daily basis, you'll inevitably encounter resistance. That resistance may initially appear as excuses—about how busy you are, how little time you have, et cetera. When you dig deeper, you'll discover emotions related to your excuses—maybe it's guilt over taking time for yourself or worry that your child will need you if you're always available at the "right" moments. As you dig even deeper, you'll discover that at the root of it all, there's a limiting belief, or several, that is the true foundation of your resistance.

I had one of these aha moments during a family vacation in Florida about five years ago. We'd come for the sunshine and the sand, but for once Walt Disney World was a drive away instead of a plane ride away. When a family member asked me if we were planning on taking the kids to Disney World, I paused. We'd set a budget and agreed to stick to it. I knew I needed to honor that promise; but in that moment of hesitation, I was overcome by a huge wave of guilt and shame. *What kind of mother would deprive her children of Disney World?* Suddenly racked with guilt, I lashed out defensively, angry at my relative for "making" me feel this way. "Are *you* going to pay for it?" I shot back.

Hearing my sharp tone of voice, I left the room to take a little time to myself. How had my good vacation mood been so suddenly disrupted? Why did a Disney vacation suddenly feel like the only important thing I could do for my children? Asking myself questions like these, I realized that I'd been subconsciously telling myself (yet another) story about what a "good" mother does. Aware of how those stories had misled me in the past, I knew that feeling like I "should" take the kids to Disney World was a sure sign that I shouldn't. The story I'd been telling myself was about what I thought other people expected of me, not what *I* thought was best.

In the end, we stuck to our budget and relaxed, knowing that we were vacationing within our means. While I "deprived" my children of Disney World, we enjoyed the sun and surf, played games, and had a memorable, fun-filled two weeks in a house we rented at no cost from a home-swapping website.

Because I was able to notice the story I'd been telling myself—that a "good" mother would take her children to Disney World, no matter the cost—I didn't let it dictate my actions. As a result, that particular story did not create additional debt. In the end it impacted my mood for a few hours and no more. That, however, is the exception. Most of the time, the stories we tell ourselves control our lives for much longer and with noticeable and long-lasting consequences.

"I Have to Do It All"

When Stephanie first came to me, she was at her wit's end. With two jobs and multiple school-aged children, she'd spent years taking on most of the burden of parenting, in part because her husband had begun insisting that he'd never wanted so many children. Exhausted and overwhelmed, she felt like she was finally ready to begin speaking her truth to him.

After keeping her growing resentment inside for so long, their "talking" began with her yelling. While fighting and blaming is not always constructive, it is sometimes a necessary part of the process. I urged her to let it out, and above all to keep going, to *not* give up, even when she felt like she was messing everything up. For years she'd worn herself dim, telling herself the story that she "had to" be everything to her children. After holding all of those emotions in, she needed to release her frustration, anger, and exhaustion before she would be able to communicate constructively.

As time went on, she sometimes yelled and other times showed up apologizing for the yelling she'd been doing. The process felt awkward, even embarrassing, but she persevered. As weeks turned into months, she and her husband began to break through and communicate. About six months into my mastery program, she emailed me. Her husband was spending more time with her and their children. Instead of showing up passive-aggressively, as she had in the past, she was showing up differently with him and realizing that when she was kind, her husband was kind in return. Her oldest child had even thanked her and her husband for getting along better.

This is the kind of change I repeatedly see in clients who are brave enough to see their own stories for what they are—deeply rooted limiting beliefs—and write new ones, no matter how messy, imperfect, and chaotic the change process feels.

Do Any of These Beliefs Resonate?

The stories we tell ourselves are often subconscious beliefs we are taught and then internalize at a deep level. Since we don't consciously recognize them as beliefs—they often feel like the truth—we don't typically talk about them. As a result, we often don't realize how many others are suffering from similarly limiting beliefs.

It's important for you to know that you're *not* suffering alone. There are numerous limiting beliefs that I see often in the women I coach. Here are some of the more common ones:

- Giving to myself means taking away from others, especially my child(ren).

- I need to provide my child(ren) with stimulating experiences, no matter their age or how exhausted I am.

- I have to be perpetually available to my child(ren) because I'm the only one who will care for them the right way.

- If I'm not attentive to my child(ren) at all times, they will suffer.

- I need to help my child(ren) process every emotion. Otherwise, they will suffer.

- If I'm not giving my child(ren) the best of everything—clothing, education, birthdays, experiences, opportunities—they will never be their best, and it will be all my fault.

- My child(ren) need to be stimulated and engaged at all times.

- Screen time will undermine my child(ren)'s development.

- If I can't always provide organic, nutritious, "perfect" food, my child(ren)'s health will suffer, and it will be my fault.

Why We Hold On to Our Old, Limiting Beliefs

It was so clear that my limiting beliefs about motherhood weren't serving me. For years, I felt physically sick—exhausted, nauseated on and off, and always so, so tired. Why did I ignore my body's signals for so long? Why did I resist looking at the stories I told myself about what I could and couldn't do, should and shouldn't be so much that it took almost dying for me to show up and do the work of taking on new beliefs?

I wish I could say I was unusual in this way, that my clients jump at the opportunity to recognize and rewrite their own limiting beliefs. Unfortunately, most of us don't. We know something has to give and change needs to happen, but often it takes crisis, or near crisis, for us to be willing to acknowledge that the stories we've been telling ourselves are just beliefs, not truths.

Why are we so attached to beliefs that clearly hurt us and downgrade our lives?

It's a big, complicated question, but here's what I've learned so far: Our worth, as women, has always been tied to our ability to serve and nurture others. Caretaking has long been our primary role and we have fulfilled it well. We are nurturers. We are givers. In this, there's a lot of good, but also the belief that we only matter when we're focused on others.

According to that way of thinking, it's shameful for us, as women, to take care of ourselves and feel good because it means we're not giving all of our time and energy to others. Even now, even today, a woman who feels good and is thriving in one or many parts of her life is judged as selfish or self-centered—even conceited. If that woman happens to be a mother, she's often criticized even more harshly. If she's not spending every waking second caring for her children, our culture says, she's not fulfilling her duties as a "good" mother.

This stigma around us, as women, spending our own time and energy to care for ourselves weighs on us all. I still struggle with my own shame around feeling good, being successful, and living my dream. I still self-sabotage sometimes when my body and my energy are at their peak, resorting to eating chips that make me feel sick afterward when whole foods would make me feel amazing. Even after all of the personal development work I've done, I am not immune to the limiting belief that I, as a woman, should feel ashamed of feeling good.

When we justify our self-sacrifice—that fiftieth yoga class we skipped to play Legos—by asserting that giving to ourselves means taking away from others, we're stuck in a scarcity mindset. Scarcity says that there's never enough of anything to go around, so we must self-sacrifice in order to help others. The actual truth is that the Universe is naturally oriented toward abundance. While there is a lot of pain and suffering in this world, our success contributes to others' success; when any one of us rises, we show other women that they, too, can succeed. By dimming our light in order to "save" or "protect" others, we're accomplishing neither of those goals. Instead of giving others the inspiration to rise, we're modeling self-sacrifice and validating others who are also self-sacrificing. Scarcity creates more scarcity, and abundance creates more abundance.

When we do the work of examining our limiting beliefs and rewriting our stories in ways that allow us to feel good, we give more women permission to do the same for themselves.

Daring to Stand Out

"Fitting in is about assessing a situation and becoming who you need to be to be accepted. Belonging, on the other hand, doesn't require us to change who we are; it requires us to be who we are."
Brené Brown, *The Gifts of Imperfection*

A married mother of two young children, Rhonda was determined to realize her dream of owning and growing her own business. She'd always gravitated toward sales and loved how engaging the sales process had always felt to her. Above all, she wanted to feel and be her best for herself and her two young children, as well as her husband. However, as her business became more successful, some of her relatives began criticizing her for her success, claiming that she thought she was better than them. Their remarks hurt Rhonda deeply. She didn't want to have to choose between her dreams and her family, but the more she showed up for her own desires, the more these family members sought her out to say unkind things to her.

It was a difficult process to navigate. These were her relatives, but would she continue to allow them to control her decisions and limit her happiness? Their harsh comments were a reflection of their discomfort with her decisions, not her own discomfort. Should she prioritize their judgments and desires over her own?

Sometimes, when we choose to honor what we think and what we want over what others want for us, we may receive critical, even harsh and unwarranted, feedback from others. In other words, by using our time and energy to take care of ourselves instead of others, we risk being judged and potentially also excluded from groups and opportunities.

This can be a deeply uncomfortable position to be in, but it's also a relatively common one. When this does happen, we have to step back and focus on belonging instead of fitting in. When we seek to belong, we look for people who see us and accept us for who we truly are. This gives us freedom to evolve, strive, rise, fall, and shine without giving up these relationships. The people we belong with don't judge us harshly for succeeding, failing, or staying where we are. They see us, appreciate us, and allow us to belong as we are. However, when we try to fit in, we have to change ourselves in order to be part of a group.

To fit in with her family, Rhonda would have had to shut down her business and play small in her life in order to make her family comfortable with her choices again. The problem, of course, was that while her relatives might have been more willing to accept her, she would have felt miserable. Realizing this, Rhonda chose to continue pursuing her dream.

How Our Limiting Beliefs Hide in Plain Sight

As I've mentioned, because our limiting beliefs look and sound like the truth, we're often unaware of how much influence they're having over us and our decisions. What follows is an example of how a limiting belief might manifest in the ETM process.

A client connects with her desired feelings, sets up ETM, including her calendar, and schedules in an hour of one-on-one time each week with each of her children. That, she reasons, will help her feel more connected, which is one of her desired feelings. However, after following her new schedule, she's still not feeling connected. Instead, she's feeling exhausted and overwhelmed, which is how she's been feeling for a long time.

When I probe into why she's still not feeling connected, it becomes clear that her desire for connection has nothing to do with her children. She already spends a lot of time with them. What she's craving is connection with herself, her husband, and her friends; she's craving time with other adults. However, she resists the idea of using that time for herself, her husband, and her friends because she feels guilty for "depriving" her children. Underneath all of this is her limiting belief that taking care of herself is equal to taking away from her children; that she's not allowed to satisfy her own needs and desires because taking care of her children has to take up more of her time and energy.

That's how our limiting beliefs work—they operate in plain sight, but also manage to stay hidden by looking like what we should do or appearing to be the truth.

Noticing Your Limiting Beliefs

Recently, I received an email from a listener of my podcast, *Mom Is In Control*, that subtly highlighted how limiting beliefs can show up in our lives when we're unaware of them, and also how powerfully and quickly we can transform our experience once we see and change them.

Dear Heather,

I want to tell you just how you are changing my life. I wish every woman would listen to your podcast.

Last school year, mornings went like this . . . I'd squeeze in a workout in the basement before waking the kids, then spend the next hour, still in sweaty clothes, getting the kids up to search for socks, underwear, favorite jeans. Then we'd go to the breakfast table, and I'd madly pack lunches and clean the kitchen—yes, still sweaty and quite uncomfortable.

Once everyone had gone off to school, I'd finally exhale, as if I'd just run a marathon, and take a shower, already exhausted from my day. I'd say to myself, "At least I got twenty minutes on the bike, at least I took care of myself before everyone else." Giving myself a pat on the back, I'd dive into laundry, cleaning, maybe, just maybe, getting to my computer to do work by 11:00.

But, thanks to you, I've been asking myself repeat-edly, *How do I want to feel?* I've also been sharing what I'm learning with my husband, aka Carefree Carl, who never did "get" how much I was doing in the morning.

Today went differently. I awoke, took a deep breath, and spent a few minutes stretching the sleep out of my bones before getting up to get on my treadmill. Looking around at my bedroom, I asked myself again, *How do I want to feel?* Instead of rushing through my workout, I decided to try finishing the laundry before waking the kids. When my kids woke up, I already had the chore I hate the most... *done!*

Next I discovered that, without me knowing it, my husband had had the kids pack their lunches the night before. *Score!*

The kids came down to breakfast on their own, without reminders. They were calm and smiling... why? We'd made the time the night before to lay out clothes. When they left the house, the chores were done and the kitchen was clean, so I did a *forty-five-minute* workout. I ran ten miles, when I usually only have time for three.

By 10:00, I was at the computer, getting work done, so instead of doing that extra hour of work tonight after the kids' bedtime, I'm going to watch a TV show. Woohoo!

The icing on our day started with asking myself, *How do I want to feel after school?*

Last year, I would dread 3:00. The kids would come home from school and, outside of homework, it was a five-hour battle over electronics, lying around, making messes... Instead, today I packed up some towels and a football and announced that we were going to the park. I wanted to feel the fresh air and enjoy the perfect autumn weather.

Both kids whined for a hot second before hopping in the car. They ran and played and recharged while I took a nap. It was awesome. When we came home, my teenager dove right into his homework with no reminders or complaints. This has never happened before. Homework has been a daily battle since second grade.

What a glorious way to start the week! I feel better than I have in a really long time.

I love you, Heather, for all you have taught me and my family.

Thank you.

To help you see the limiting beliefs that this listener—we'll call her Jess—was able to rewrite, let's dissect her email (which has been edited slightly for length, but the meaning of which remains largely the same).

Subconscious Story #1: I'm exercising first, which means I'm prioritizing self-care. First, when she discusses how mornings went last year, she talks about how she put herself "first" by squeezing in her workout. The subconscious story there was, *I'm exercising first, which means I'm prioritizing self-care.*

I see this very literal approach to self-care in so many clients. With no regard for how they're feeling, they add self-care basics, like daily movement or drinking water, to their to-do lists and tick off the extra boxes each week, completely ignoring the fact that activities that bring them joy and contribute to their health and well-being should *not* be jammed between work and cleaning!

When Jess used her time differently, she was able to exercise in a way that *felt* good to her.

Subconscious Story #2: There's never enough time. Beneath this story about going through the motions of practicing self-care, which in her case meant frantically jumping on the treadmill for less time than she wanted, she also seems to have had a story around never having enough time. As she experienced, however, when we plan, use our time better, and seek support, we don't just have enough time, we sometimes have extra time to relax.

Subconscious Story #3: I need to follow my usual routine, no matter how I feel. This is a less significant story, but still an important one. Before taking into account how she was feeling, she made a point of sticking to the same routine every day, even though it wasn't working.

When we look at routine this rigidly, we put a lot of unnecessary and unproductive pressure on ourselves. When instead we consider how we want to feel, we can find new solutions, like Jess did, that align with our desired feelings.

Subconscious Story #4: Carefree Carl doesn't "get" how much I do (and won't step up to support me). For years Jess had been telling herself that her husband was essentially too clueless to see how much she was doing. However, she hadn't ever told him how underappreciated or overwhelmed she felt. When she finally did speak up, he sprang into action and got the kids to make their lunches the night before.

Too many of us spend years waiting for our partners, friends, and family to acknowledge, understand, and support us when instead we should actively communicate our thoughts, feelings, needs, and desires.

Subconscious Story #5: "Have-tos" always need to come before "want-tos." Since our joy and pleasure are seen as shameful, we prioritize them last. Instead of giving ourselves opportunities to feel good, we dive into our have-tos first. Unfortunately, our have-to lists only get longer, so the more we do, the more there is to do. This habit of pushing our joy and pleasure to the bottom of our priority list becomes so ingrained, we often carry it over into our parenting, causing us to parent in ways that emphasize have-tos over want-tos and obligation over joy.

When Jess challenged this belief around prioritizing have-tos (schoolwork) over want-tos (playing outside) by taking her kids to the park first, they were better able to focus on homework afterward. When we feel better, we do better. By being more flexible and fitting in fun before homework, Jess created more joy and ease in their weekday afternoon.

OF COURSE, Jess's email is just one piece of her larger story, and what she shared reflects only one set of limiting beliefs. We each have our own limiting beliefs and they can manifest in a lot of different ways. When you're practicing ETM, it's important to start recognizing your own subconscious limiting beliefs because they'll influence how you navigate ETM and what kind of resistance you experience as you begin to practice it.

As you begin to see your limiting beliefs—about what you're "allowed" to do and be, about how you're "allowed" to use your time and energy, and more—you'll also encounter your big emotions.

Feeling Your Big Emotions

Anger. Sadness. Regret. Guilt. Fear. Shame.

When you start to practice filling your cup first—tending to your needs and desires before others'—you'll inevitably face a lot of big emotions that you may at first assume mean that you're doing something wrong. In fact, you're growing, and in that process, feeling emotions you've been avoiding for a long time.

When I began to practice ETM myself, I felt guilt around not doing "enough" for my children. I also felt fear around being seen as a coach and in my business. I also experienced anger around being pushed beyond my former limits. Numerous times, I was forced to feel my big emotions and throughout, I turned to The Work, a practice created by Byron Katie. On her website she defines it this way:

The Work is a Practice

Every time you do The Work you are becoming enlightened to who and what you are, the true nature of being. To question what you believe is an amazing gift to give yourself, and you can have it all the days of your life. The answers are always inside you, just waiting to be heard.

According to Katie's methodology, the first step of The Work is getting in touch with what you're feeling by letting it out, unedited. Then you focus on the main thought behind your big emotion and ask yourself four questions:

1. Is it true?
2. Can you absolutely know that it's true?
3. How do you react (what happens) when you believe that thought?
4. Who would you be without the thought?

For example, if you're angry because your child won't listen to you, and in the heat of the moment you think, *My child never listens to me!* you would then ask yourself:

1. Is it true that he never listens to me?
2. Can I absolutely know that it's true that he never listens to me?
3. How do I react (what happens) when I believe the thought, *He never listens to me*?
4. Who would I be without the thought, *He never listens to me*?

My own life and so many of my clients' lives have been transformed by practicing The Work. One client even told me her husband thought she was taking anti-anxiety medication! She was so much calmer that he couldn't imagine any other reason.

Get Byron Katie's Worksheets

For a deeper understanding of The Work, as well as free downloadable copies of Byron Katie's Worksheets, visit her website at thework.com.

From Emotion to Action

One of the reasons The Work is so important is because our big emotions can be so overwhelming, they paralyze us. Instead of taking the action we need to take to feel the way we want to feel, we freeze and do nothing, or go back to ignoring our own desires.

Making changes and doing new things can feel challenging, but that's not a reason to hesitate. The resistance you feel around doing new things is an indication that it's time for you to propel yourself into action—even when it doesn't feel right or easy or natural. When in doubt, take action. Even the "wrong" action will bring you closer to how you want to feel. Instead of resorting to inaction, force yourself to do something, anything, that creates movement inside you and your life.

As you practice ETM, just go ahead and do what your calendar is telling you to do. As you move forward, keep asking, *How do I want to feel? Is this activity/pursuit/task helping me to feel how I want to feel?* You can only answer that question by taking action; anything less is guesswork. After taking the action, ask yourself if it has helped you to feel your desired feelings. Over time, one action by one, you find your way, forge your own path, and manifest your desired feelings.

NOW THAT we've looked at the essential steps of the journey, let's look at how showing up and taking courageous action can transform your life.

14

Fearful but Not Afraid

MY HEART THUMPING in my chest, sweat dripping from my pores, I couldn't avoid the primal fear coursing through my body. The months leading up to this moment hadn't felt easy, safe, or familiar. Finally, the big day, the big moment, was here. I *had to* walk onstage. I *had to* perform. I was here to inspire, motivate, and connect—but would I be good enough? Could I ever be that good?

Terrified, I walked toward center stage, flashing my best fake smile, wanting nothing more than to run and hide.

Just don't crap your pants, Heather.

During the previous few days, I'd been extra mindful of how I was fueling my body, cutting back on caffeine and managing my anxiety so I could feel in control of my body at this exact moment.

The event was a speaker slam—a competitive in-person speaking event. I'd been afraid to even apply, which I'd seen as a message from the Universe that I *had to* apply, specifically because my resistance felt *that* intense. Just to be accepted as a speaker, I'd had to drive an eight-hour round trip two separate times to attend mandatory events in Toronto. I'd also had to postpone a family vacation by a few days to fit it all into my schedule. Getting accepted had taken weeks, and since receiving that first yes, I'd invested hours and hours in writing, rewriting, and memorizing my speech with the help of a speaker coach.

Throughout the process, I'd done everything I'd been afraid of, including showing up for every part of the process. For once, if my performance was disappointing, I wouldn't be able to blame my lack of preparation; whatever happened, I'd have to take responsibility for my results.

And here I was, about to begin. Looking at the audience, feeling the heat and light all around me, I took a breath. "I remember walking out of the hospital after my husband and I were given the news..." I began.

Feeling your fear and taking action anyway can change your life. If you do it often enough, it *will* change your life—but you have to show up. You have to do things that feel uncomfortable. You have to take action that feels too big or too scary or too much or too little of... [fill in the blank]. Ladies, it's time to stop waiting for the "right" time, "right" feeling, or "right" amount of money or energy. Courage means being scared shitless and doing it anyway.

It's time to crap your pants, ladies.

As we come to the last part of this process, we'll take a closer look at what it really means to feel your fear and take action anyway. We'll also revisit some important principles to keep in mind as you continue taking courageous action and practicing ETM.

Get Ready to Be Uncomfortable

Feel your fear and take action anyway—it's something we say and quickly agree with. We know it's what we're supposed to do, but when we're in the thick of our own fear, stunned by its sheer force and intensity, we panic and run away or freeze. Before we know it, we resort to old limiting behaviors, and we default, often subconsciously, to old beliefs that keep us from feeling how we want to feel and living how we want to live. "Feel your fear and take action anyway"—words that are easy to say, but a challenge to live by.

On Overcoming

It's interesting looking back, especially at this moment in time. Except for periodic weekends at my dad's house, I grew up in a trailer park and became a low-income single mother on welfare by age eighteen. Throughout, I felt unworthy, alone, and unsupported—the "not smart," undeserving kid whose future had been prematurely labeled dim. Determined to prove my worth and yearning for proof that I belonged somewhere, as I got older, I gave to everyone who "needed" me except myself. For years I used self-sacrifice as my armor, hoping to protect myself from the pain that had long been simmering inside me. I tried to prove that I was enough even as I was making myself smaller and smaller still. As a white-skinned, able-bodied woman, there's no denying that I have benefited from privilege. This journey would have been significantly more challenging had I been the target of systemic bias and oppression. And yet, none of it felt easy.

What Is Fear, Really?

Fear can feel bigger than life, bigger than any one of us. That's because it's embedded in the primitive brain and our basic human survival instinct. It also shows us what needs more attention and how we need to show up next. It's one of our many faithful guides, helping to illuminate the path ahead. However, we can only figure out how to use fear as a guide if we make peace with the fact that, at least to some degree, it will always be with us.

In other words, we can only use fear to our ultimate advantage if we accept that we can never fully overcome it. For me this means:

- I may never stop being afraid of not being able to "save" people.

- I may always feel some degree of fear around being seen by more and more people.

- I may never stop wrestling with the nagging feeling of not being "enough" in some ways.

- I may always be afraid of not giving enough.

- I may always feel afraid of hurting other people's feelings.

These and other fears may be with me forever, but I can choose not to let them run my life.

What are you deeply afraid of? Which fears never seem to go away completely? Staying consciously aware of your deeper fears is an important step in realizing that they're not valid reasons to hold yourself back, avoid taking uncomfortable action, or hide or dim your light.

If you wait for the day when you're not afraid, you're waiting for a day that will never come.

Fearfully Numb

We react to fear differently at different times in our lives. Now when I'm afraid or overwhelmed by other big emotions, I tend to go numb. I feel "fine," as I often do when I'm digesting and processing discomfort, struggling to feel into what's next while trying to take courageous action in the meantime.

It's odd being in that place emotionally while also hearing from women, even on my lowest days, that they see me as someone who's brave enough to be herself, largely unedited and almost always unscripted. I assume that's because I show up as honestly as I can, trying not to pretend that everything's great when it's not. I don't want to hide my imperfections; I want to share them so that women can move their own lives forward—even when, especially when, it feels really, really uncomfortable.

Above all, I want women to know and understand that while I take courageous action often—by moving my life and business forward and by sharing some of what I'm experiencing—I never do any of it perfectly. I love being challenged and I do pursue challenges, but I also often feel fearful, ashamed, and sometimes blah or disconnected too. Taking courageous action doesn't come easily for me. It's simply a habit I committed to years ago that helps me feel some of my most deeply desired feelings: alive and energized.

I see so many women abandoning or sabotaging their own courageous action because the experience feels too confusing or too slow. These feelings of overwhelm are normal; they're all forms of resistance. Whenever you feel any kind of resistance around showing up and taking bold action, know that you're not alone. I, and so many women like you, are going through our days feeling as daunted by the intensity and raw power of our fear and our shame around being "not enough" or "too much."

The big emotions that fuel our resistance can feel like a tsunami surging inside us, like a wall we can't possibly move beyond. The thing is, though, even when our fear and our feelings of not enough-ness seem insurmountable, they're still just feelings. They're never stronger or bigger than us; they only feel that way sometimes. One of the reasons I continually nudge myself toward my brave zone—that place where I'm deep in my emotional shit and feeling resistance but taking action anyway—is because each time I'm in it, I become a little braver. Every time I put myself in that vulnerable, messy, uncomfortable place, I'm reminded that I can do it again next time.

Understanding How You Respond to Fear

How does fear-induced resistance show up for you?

We each respond to fear differently. I tend to resort to sleeping, feeling low energy and depressed, and sometimes also eating a bag of chips. However, when I finally get over myself long enough to take courageous action, I feel so much better that I can't remember why I resisted taking action in the first place.

Creating a new and more constructive relationship with fear starts with creating more awareness around how fear tends to show up and sabotage your momentum.

How do you react to fear?

Do you say "I'm good" when you're really not?

Do you default to the excuse of "I don't know what I want"?

Do you use excuses about your kids needing you, you not being "good" with technology, not having enough time, money, energy, or other?

Do you disrespect your own time and energy by not planning ahead, setting boundaries, or prioritizing your own desires?

Do you nitpick in order to avoid taking imperfect action? (Fear, shame, and perfectionism are closely intertwined.)

Do you become hyper-critical, impatient, or quick to anger?
All of these reactions are ways of deflecting the emotional
turmoil and fear you're feeling around taking courageous action.
By noticing how resistance tends to show up for you, you can
catch yourself more easily and more often, and then take courageous action in spite of your fear.

When you feel resistance and discomfort, keep moving. It's the
only way to benefit from the Law of Inspired Action.

The Law of Inspired Action

I'd been working with Rachel for about a year when she
attended one of my live events. She'd recently given birth to
her fifth child, who was just weeks old. She'd made so much
progress already. During the previous year, which had been
our first year working together, she'd addressed health issues
by changing her food and exercise to improve her physical and
mental energy. She and her husband had also begun communicating about finances and were cultivating deeper trust as
a result. With my guidance, she'd also begun to view her children's behavior as a language and was yelling less as a result.
Having undergone so much transformation, she was ready to
cultivate her creativity and take her photography business to
the next level. As she put it, "When I'm creative, I'm better at
everything in my life."

Soon after the pandemic hit in the spring of 2020, Rachel
really began to walk her talk. She pivoted soon after lockdown
started, using video technology to conduct virtual photo
shoots that kept her business afloat and allowed her to remain

connected to her creativity. This is the magic that unfolds when you begin to get out of your own way and make your desired feelings a non-negotiable priority.

When I step back and look at why women like Rachel are able to manifest such powerful results with ETM, I notice some common themes. Without exception, they make an ongoing commitment to their dreams and desires. On a deeper level, they believe in their Big Why and become invested in the bigger vision they've created for their life. As a result, they're more willing to step out of their comfort zones and into their brave zones. No matter how scared they feel, they take action, even when they feel unsettled and unsure; even when the excuses they could use, such as a pandemic, seem incredibly valid.

Over and over again, women like Rachel follow the Law of Inspired Action, which is one of the twelve spiritual laws. The law states that we have to take continual action that brings us closer to our desires in order to realize them.

Attracting what you desire happens in proportion to how often you take courageous action. Now and always, action is where the magic happens.

Revisiting Your Big Why

Sometimes taking the next courageous action means reviewing and recommitting to your Big Why. (For a refresher, see "Finding Your Big Why" in Chapter 11, page 181.)

What is your Big Why? Does it still feel authentic? Are you feeling called toward a new or deeper sense of purpose? Don't hesitate to revise your Big Why as you evolve.

Remember, your Big Why should be for you and about you. It's your reason for showing up to co-create your desires, and it should inspire you immediately, automatically, and instinctively. This isn't a time to worry about how others might judge you or your Big Why. This is a time to focus only on what you want and why you want it.

Each woman's Big Why is unique. Sometimes it may feel like a profound sense of being destined for "something bigger" or a desire to break a multi-generational family pattern or give back to humanity and our planet. Over time this deeper, broader sense of purpose may develop. For example, if you start the process wanting to model empowered motherhood, you might later connect with a desire to model empowered womanhood. Whatever your Big Why may be at any given time, it's important to keep checking in with it, making sure it's still compelling enough to draw you forward, even when taking action on it feels profoundly uncomfortable.

If you're unclear on your Big Why or whether it still feels authentic, try taking a new and different kind of courageous action. As you take more action, you'll gain more clarity around how your Big Why is or isn't changing.

On Taking Courageous Action

As you take courageous action, keep these basic principles in mind. They can have a huge impact on your ability to create sustainable change.

Thinking positively is 90 percent of the challenge. When I tell myself I can't do something, I can't. When I tell myself I can do something, I can. In my experience, thoughts determine 90 percent of your ability to take courageous action.

Do you believe you can take the next courageous action? Do you believe that you and your desires matter? Do you believe you have the power to create change?

Taking courageous action isn't about always getting the results you're hoping for, and it isn't meant to feel safe or simple. However, if you're constantly saying mean things to yourself, your first courageous action should be to transform your self-talk. Feeling afraid is normal, but constantly telling yourself you're not enough or don't deserve the life you desire will eventually prevent you from taking the courageous action necessary to create the changes you desire.

Don't worry about believing if you can manifest your full vision of the life you desire; that's a process. All you have to believe is that you can take the next courageous action, even when you feel afraid.

Your thoughts are the engine behind every courageous action you do or don't take. As you practice ETM, continue to notice them.

Finding an accountability partner is paramount. Who's keeping you accountable for taking courageous action? Even those of us who are introverted tend to be more willing and able to take courageous action when someone is keeping us accountable. Find a trusted friend, coach, or mentor who will check in regularly and be sure you're staying on track with practicing ETM and taking courageous action.

Creating space for yourself allows you to make progress that's sustainable. While having a physical space to focus is important, it's far more important to give yourself time-related space to figure out what works for you. When I work with clients on making a plan, we typically plan in ninety-day segments. By creating that space to realize goals and outcomes—and get tripped up, make mistakes, and so on in the process—you allow yourself to move through your process at a sustainable pace. Remember, you're going for progress, not perfection. I'd much rather you make 10 percent or even 1 percent progress consistently than for you to push yourself to move at breakneck speed and then quit from exhaustion and feelings of overwhelm.

Assigning specific actions to each of your desires facilitates progress. It's so important to commit to specific actions related to realizing the outcomes you desire. For example, if one of your desires is to stop yelling at your children, that may be a sign that you need more quiet time to digest your own thoughts and feelings. To meet that need, schedule in daily journaling time where you can dump your thoughts on the page and get more centered in how you want to feel. Or, if you feel rushed all the time and want to feel calm, say no to an event that no longer aligns with your desired feelings and schedule in a walk or meditation time instead. Focus on each desired feeling and pinpoint specific actions that will help you feel that way. If those actions don't produce the feeling you desire, try a different action.

Using mind mapping as a planning tool enables you to tap into your intuitive, creative side. I'm a big fan of mind mapping, which allows you to connect your desired feelings and outcomes with actions. It's an intuitive way of planning that allows you to be both creative and practical. To find resources on how to use mind mapping, go to dyingtobeagoodmother.com.

Mindset Shifts and Reminders

As you and your life change, your days, as well your desires, will inevitably evolve. As those changes become apparent, these mindset tips can help to keep you moving forward:

When you feel triggered, get curious and keep taking action. We all get triggered sometimes. Rather than hiding—whether by avoiding taking courageous action, using excuses to justify not showing up, or something else—try to get curious. There's no shame in being triggered; we all experience it at different times and for different reasons. By giving yourself permission to be curious about your triggers, you can figure out what's really bothering you.

So often, our external triggers are actually internal. For example, when our children push our buttons, they're usually pressing on parts of us we haven't yet fully healed. In other words, we're triggered because of wounds we've been holding on to that have little to do with what our children are doing or saying.

By being a detective and looking for the real reason you're feeling triggered, you can discover the true source of your pain and begin to heal it.

Accept that failure is universal and inevitable—and a great way to learn. Failure is a fact of life that none of us can escape. Rather than hiding in shame or viewing failure as a final judgment on your worthiness, try to see it as a learning opportunity.

When failure strikes, ask yourself, *What did I overlook? What did I not expect to happen that then did? What would I do differently next time?* Use failure as an opportunity, process your disappointment and other emotions, and then get up and try again.

Know that ETM will feel messy, and that's okay. Perfection is a myth, which also means there's no perfect way to practice ETM. At times it's going to feel very messy. At other times you'll feel out of sorts and out of sync. That's all normal. Reach out for help when you need, and know that living in the mess of your own evolution is part of the human experience. If you keep taking action toward your vision and your desires, you can and will find your groove.

Stepping into Joy

As soon as I heard my name, my jaw locked shut. I walked forward to accept my prize, but I couldn't even crack a smile. The truth was, nothing about this moment felt good.

Second place? Why second place?

Throughout the process, I'd told myself and everyone who knew about the speaker slam that I was viewing the experience as a "personal development exercise." If that had been true, wouldn't I have felt good in this moment? I'd grown enormously as a result of the experience. I'd faced huge resistance repeatedly and showed up consistently anyway. If growth was my goal, I'd delivered a five-star, A-plus performance. So why didn't I feel amazing accepting my prize? Why had winning second place put a damper on everything?

As I walked off the stage toward my family, Bryan was smiling. "You secretly wanted first place, didn't you?" he asked.

"No, I didn't," I replied, suddenly feeling defensive.

You should be proud of yourself, Heather. Why can't you allow yourself to feel good?

Yes, I secretly had wanted first place, and I'd missed it by one point. One! In the end, my actual growing edge hadn't been in facing my fear and showing up before and during the event, it was allowing myself to feel joy afterward—even without a first-place prize.

Brené Brown has famously said, "Joy is probably the most vulnerable emotion we experience. We're afraid that if we allow ourselves to feel it, we'll get blindsided by disaster or disappointment. That's why in moments of real joy, many of us dress-rehearse tragedy." In this case I wasn't dress-rehearsing for tragedy, but I was downplaying my achievement and tamping down on the joy I could have been feeling. As is usual for me, it felt safer to be dissatisfied and disappointed at not having won first place than to celebrate and feel proud of winning second.

I do this often, even now, even after surviving cancer and building the business I'd always dreamed of owning. Even today, after so many years of proving myself in my brave zone, I still struggle with feeling joy.

I'm not alone in this. I see so many clients, friends, and family members backing away from opportunities to feel good. We can do better, ladies. Taking courageous action and living our fullest, biggest lives will start to feel punishing if we don't let ourselves feel joy.

It takes incredible courage to feel good, but it's also why we're here. It's why we show up to do this work—because there's joy and it's available to us in almost limitless abundance if we're courageous enough to feel it.

Let's go there together. Let's take big, bold, courageous action toward our desires and actually allow ourselves to feel good about how we're showing up.

What Are You Waiting For?

You can do amazing things if you're willing to feel uncomfortable and take action anyway. If you're already putting the self-development principles and practices I've laid out into practice, congratulations! Keep moving forward. Keep taking imperfect action. Keep making progress without expecting perfection.

If you haven't yet implemented the steps I've laid out, go back to the beginning of Part III. Now—not later, not tomorrow—is the time to start implementing the process I use with clients to create amazing results.

It's go time, ladies! I'm ready to stretch and expand and go for it, cheering on your every step as you do the same. Will you join me?

Conclusion

DEAR HEATHER,

Do you remember when you decided not to die?

You heard a whisper, "Don't let go, you have a big purpose here." The voice felt so much bigger than you.

You were in grade nine. You asked to go to the washroom. Walking down the hall, tears streaming down your face, you were making a plan to leave your body. Being human felt too painful. Back then, it all felt so unbearable.

Walking back to class, you wiped your eyes and put on a mask. You know the mask; "fake it till you make it." Isn't that what they say to do?

Needless to say, you stayed in your body that night.

Then, three years later, you saw those two parallel lines on your first pregnancy test.

Something profound shifted inside you then. You were terrified. You felt alone, unseen, and misunderstood. But still, you decided to stay here. There was finally someone to live for. It was just the beginning.

All along I've been here guiding you, sending you hints and whispers, bringing you back home.

It's me, Heather, your body.

I will always be here to tell you when something is off. I will always nudge you when you need more rest or more movement. I forgive you for how you've treated me. I won't ever leave you. I am your constant, the home you keep returning to for comfort and energy, love and support.

By now, things have changed within you and your life. And I have something different, something kind of big, to ask of you.

But first, think back on the girl you once were. Spiritually, mentally, emotionally, and physically, you're light-years from where you used to be. You have stepped into leadership in your life and your business, as a woman and a mother. You have transformed and you have grown. Particularly since cancer, you have also pushed yourself through such deep discomfort. It's been incredibly intense, even grueling, but inspiring—and fulfilling too.

You have come so far, Heather. Yet still, you are you. Always you.

Now, at long last, you get to share your wisdom and daring with other women who need your help to find their way out of their dark places. That is not new, yet your bigger vision is still fresh, and in many ways, just coming into its true fullness.

You are ready for this next level of being seen and heard. Staying where you are would mean hiding. It would be a form of soul death, and who knows what after that.

You're scared, I know, but I'm here. I see you and I hear you. I feel your passion, your resilience, your power. You are a change-maker, and in spite of what you may tell yourself sometimes, you are prepared for what's to come.

But I need you to do something for you, for us. It may sound simple, but you and I both know how profoundly you, and so many of the women you work with, resist this.

Are you ready? Because I'm asking you, but I'm also telling you—you *must* do this. It's important. It's your lifeline; it's every woman's lifeline. You must grab it and never fully let go.

It's the good feelings, Heather. It's joy. I need you to welcome them and hold on to them. Always.

I'm demanding a lot of you, I know, especially when so many are suffering.

Still, you must lean in (just a little each day) to make yourself stronger. So I can be stronger. So we can all be stronger—as women, as a community, and as a world struggling to find its way back to love and light.

Please, whatever you do, fuel me, fuel *us*, with your love.

Are you listening to me? I need you to really listen to me. I'm asking you to let go of more layers of resistance so your bigger purpose can come into being inside and all around you.

It's time for you, and for all women, to let go of that next layer of "not enough-ness."

To release more fear, more doubt, and your ongoing need to struggle in order to "prove" your worth.

You don't need to prove your worth. You are enough. You always have been.

Do you hear me? I'm asking you to *feel* it all—the resistance and the good feelings too.

Will you finally allow yourself to celebrate who you are? To bask in the glow of getting through so much? To feel, really *feel*, all you are and all you've done and are doing?

Do you dare to let yourself feel *that* good? Can you let go of the shame and the endless pull to downplay and devalue yourself?

Will you dare to feel your wins, even when you get second place?

Because all I've been asking you for these many years . . . is to be loved.

Will you love me, Heather? Will you?

xo,

Heather

Acknowledgments

I **WROTE A BOOK!** And I definitely didn't get here alone. The stubborn, creative words and ideas trapped inside my mind, body, and soul wanted to be birthed but needed some guidance, healing, and a whole lot of "sit your ass down and get shit done, Heather" moments.

I first need to thank Wyndham Wood. Without you, there would be no book. Your patience, persistence, questions, and detective work pulled every story out of me. You took a stand for what I wanted to run away from. You carefully crafted my Heather-isms and organized my thoughts. You taught me what true creative collaboration looks like, and I am forever grateful for your love of writing and your willingness to kick my ass. We are a match made in heaven.

Richelle Fredson, it was love at first sight. A rare gem with more gems in her back pocket. A keeper who's guaranteed to make you laugh.

I would also like to acknowledge those I know and do not know who have assisted and supported the writing and publication of *Dying to Be a Good Mother*.

To the doctors—special shout-outs to Dr. H and Dr. Valero— and the nurses, healers, scientists, cancer survivors, and those who have come before me who have dedicated their lives to healing disease and telling their stories.

To John, for giving me the greatest gift: Logan. May your soul be at peace. I'll take it from here.

To my bonus moms, Wendy and Elaine, you bathed me, rubbed my feet, fed me, calmed me down, and raised my children when I didn't have the strength. It takes a village, and I'm grateful you are part of mine.

A special thank-you to my mom, Diane. Your strength is inspiring. I wouldn't be who I am without you.

To my father, thank you for showing me how to take risks doing work that I love.

To my podcast listeners, for years you've listened to my ramblings and my Heather-isms. Without your questions, thoughts, and inspiration, this book could not exist. You've shared your intimate moments with me, and I am deeply grateful for the space we share.

Stephanie Renaud, I will never forget our Starbucks meetings back when I was a lost puppy. Your early guidance will never be forgotten. Thank you.

To Jesse and your incredible team at Page Two, your patience with me, a first-time author, has been award-winning.

To my husband, Bryan, who is the silent and steady glue who has always held me together and never let go. Since the beginning, you've accepted all parts of me. I'm so grateful I gave you my email address when you asked for my phone number fourteen years ago.

And last but certainly not least, my children: Logan, Calvin, and Felix. You've given me life, taught me how to laugh, and inspired me to trust myself. I hope when you look back on your childhood, you feel safe, loved, and accepted.

About the Author

HEATHER CHAUVIN is a leadership coach who helps ambitious, overwhelmed women conquer their fears and become leaders at work and at home.

Drawing from her professional experience as a social worker and her life experience raising three boys, Heather created a signature approach to help her clients create and enjoy sustainability, profitability, and ease in business and life.

She is the host of the *Mom Is In Control* podcast, where she reveals her most vulnerable truths about womanhood, marriage, parenting, living through stage four cancer, and running a successful business without burning out. *Dying to Be a Good Mother* is her first book.

When Heather isn't busy driving her boys to hockey practice, you can find her curled up on the couch next to her husband, planning their next family adventure.

Learn more about Heather and her programs at heather chauvin.com.

CPSIA information can be obtained
at www.ICGtesting.com
Printed in the USA
BVHW072144220323
660979BV00001B/2

9 781774 580226